Schizophrenia:
A mother's story

*This book is dedicated to my
youngest son
Christian John Wakefield
and to sufferers of mental illness
all over the world*

Schizophrenia:
A mother's story

by
Georgina Wakefield

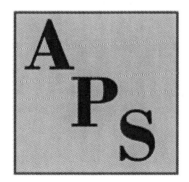

APS Publishing
The Old School, Tollard Royal, Salisbury, Wiltshire, SP5 5PW
www.apspublishing.co.uk

British Library Cataloguing in Publication Data
A catalogue record for this book is available from the British Library

Printed in the United Kingdom by Lightning Source U.K. Ltd, Milton Keynes

Contents

Acknowledgements

to Paul

This poem is dedicated to my husband Paul. He said that he did not want me to write a poem about him; he is quite a shy man, but I felt that I must. I have kept it very short.

Paul

Paul you've been my dearest friend
Ever faithful to the end
Without you I could not go on
You've shown such patience to our son

A kind, considerate, caring dad
A luxury we never had
I wonder how you learned to cope
I've shown so very little hope

But things have changed, I feel so strong
No matter what, we'll carry on
To see this journey to the end
Paul, my husband, my best friend

to Firstborn son

This poem is dedicated to my older son, Stephen. He has helped us and supported us through many bleak years. I could not have wished for a better son.

There have been times where, in my own sadness, I've forgotten that Chris isn't just our son, he's also Stephen's brother, and I'm sure that he finds it as hard as we do.

Firstborn son

Firstborn son, where do I start?
You really have the kindest heart
Supportive, patient for so long
I don't know how you've stayed so strong

You've helped me so much in nine long years
You've cooled our anger, dried our tears
When life has been so very sad
You've still supported me and dad

How well you've coped with things you've seen
At times I've felt it's all a dream

A dream from which I'll wake one day
To find the hurt has gone away

Your brother will have paid the price
He'll have a better way of life
So lets look forward to tomorrow
When hope will lift our pain and sorrow

Your brother's journey will be done
We're ever grateful first born son.

to My dearest sister

This dedication is for my sister, Christine. She has a wonderful husband, who is there for her 100%, and also her children Heidi and Neil. Her support in all these years has never faltered, even when she's been ill herself. This poem is for my dear sister whom I love dearly.

She sends Christian a few words of encouragement every week, cards and even books. He has a drawer full of them and some have even been sent from her while on holiday.

I find it hard to believe now how supportive Christine has been. The past few years have been a nightmare for her and yet, no matter what pain she's in, she still finds time for me.

My dearest sister

My dearest sister what can I say
You've been there for me from the very first day
So very close, we're two of a kind
Sometimes I swear we share the same mind

For hours on end we've talked on the phone
When I've felt scared, so lost, so alone
You've been so very ill yet you've always been there
Always supportive you've shown so much care

You'd even ring when you went away
Enquiring, "How's that boy today?"
Even when you went abroad
You'd spare me some comfort that you could afford

The countless cards you've sent to my son
Words of encouragement about battles won
You'd send him your strength via the post
I don't know which card he treasures the most

Your final gift when you said that prayer
Not a word about you, inspirational care
Now I'm convinced that prayer was heard
I've been guided word after word

Now I feel it's my time to pray
That you will receive a new heart one day
My sister who's been so strong and so true
I wonder where I would have been without you

Your prayers were answered we've been shown the way
In Kings College Chapel one rainy day
So let's look forward to a new tomorrow
With far more hope and much less sorrow.

Mum

During the past nine years, I have harboured a lot of guilt with regards to my mum. I have often felt that if my own life had been easier, I would have been able to spare much more time for her. It has been doubly hard because my sister has been so ill. At times I do not know which one I was worrying about the most. I do hope my mum understands my situation. It has been very tough on her too, as she has had all of us to worry about and that is hard to cope with as you are getting older. I love her dearly.

Mum

Mum, I've felt so guilty
I've known you've needed me
But with so many problems
I haven't been so free
To spare you time you've needed
As things have been so bad
What with Chris and Christian
It's all been very sad
But things are looking brighter
Feel more like I can cope
For my son and sister
There seems to be more hope
So let's look to tomorrow
And try hard to be strong
As the road is so precarious
That they must walk along
We'll try hard to support them
And give our very best
Life's been so unkind to them
They've got the hardest test
With you and I together
To help them on their way
We'll pass on strength and guide them
To see a better day

Jenny Lawrence of Thurrock MIND

This poem is dedicated to Jenny Lawrence and all the staff of Thurrock MIND with special thanks to Jan and Ron. I have the utmost respect for Jenny Lawrence. She has listened to my problems and talked me through them on countless occasions. Her support has been and still is second to none.

Even after losing her own son (aged 24 years) in a tragic car accident (July 22nd 1996) her support has remained 100% and she still shows the same understanding and compassion. In the beginning, she would try hard to get me to accept the situation. But to no avail. In fact, I would get very angry because I couldn't accept things. In fact, it has taken me nine years to come to terms with things.

I rang Jenny and asked her if she would mind if I included her in this book and as you can see, she agreed. A very strong lady (see *The voice* and *My son* written by Jenny Lawrence).

Jenny Lawrence of Thurrock MIND

Jenny from MIND helped me through this
So many times over the years
She'd try hard to dampen my anger
She'd ask me to dry my tears

The hardest time I remember
Happened about three years ago
My memory recalls every detail
Don't ask me how, I don't know

I rang Jenny on the Monday
As again you weren't coping so well
She asked would I ring back tomorrow
As a headache was giving her hell

She'd been to see Tina Turner
And she'd drunk a bit too much wine
I told her I'd call back tomorrow
She said "Great, tomorrow is fine"

The occasion? Her eldest son's birthday
He was 24 at the time
Her headache was self-inflicted
She'd put it all down to the wine

I rang as we'd planned on the Tuesday
Jan said "She's not here today"
"She's on leave through a family bereavement"
I just didn't know what to say

Her son had been killed in a car crash
In Horndon the previous night

I found it so hard to take in
I felt so sad for her plight

I rang MIND a few weeks later
I felt shocked when she answered the phone
I said "How can I tell you my problems,
When you've not long lost your son?"

She said "Georgie, come on now just try me
It will help me to get through
Besides it's what I'm paid for
So tell me, how are things with you?"

I was so amazed at her courage
It made me feel humble and sad
How could she keep helping others
When she'd not long lost her lad

Jenny rang me two months later to ask if Chris would like to go to the MIND
Christmas panto. He was back on the garden project after leaving work, yet
again, as it got too much for him after two weeks.

So Jenny rang to tell me
About a panto that MIND had planned
She asked if I thought Chris would go
I said "I hope so, but you'll understand"

Well Christian managed to get there
Paul and I went along with him
When Jenny Lawrence saw him
She couldn't suppress a grin

To the disco Christian was dancing
When Jenny saw him there
She threw out her arms and embraced him
So much hurt and yet so much care

Jenny I'll never forget it
And if you ask Christian nor will he
Your actions were so very selfless
To my son, my family and me

My son

Written By Jenny Lawrence

You came to us, this child so perfect
Blue eyes, Blond hair and a laugh that lit the world
We loved, nurtured and protected you
So you would be a fine man
Fate does not allow for all of this
This loss to our family
The knock that came that night

Has left a hole in our lives that will never heal
We just live with it
All our hopes and dreams for you, our son
Gone with that knock at the door
People were so kind, so very kind
Flowers cards to tell us they cared
But people go, so quiet
Not now your name mentioned in passing
We hold our dreams to our hearts
Because they are ours and we want you back
To touch your face and hear you laugh
This blond blue-eyed child, that brought us so much joy
That lived to be a man.... And then was gone.

The voice

The phone rang that day and the woman's voice said
My name is Georgie and I have a son"
That phone call was the beginning of a journey
Which has lasted for eight years
This mother, so worried about her child

"He's doing this and he's doing that
The fear in her voice with every call
It couldn't be could it Jenny
Those dreadful words, mental illness

Go here, talk, let professional people know, they will help
Was my response to this mother
Who was a voice consumed with worry and fear
It's just a phase she was told, he'll grow out of it
It! What was it?

It plagued her child every day and night
I am a mother and my heart went out, unable to really help
Just hold the voice and cry and laugh with her
Through a few good times
But an awful amount of bad

I came to know this family
Mum, dad and brother
All so scared for this child, now a man
Would he ever find a place in this world where he could cope
And the demon he lived with go away

Eventually the day came
"Schizophrenia!" the dreaded name
Georgie said it, her voice hollow with despair
Now he will get the help I said, hang in there
There's a light at the end for this man

I have watched this family fight for their beloved son
This mother who would fight the world for her child to have a life
I lost my son forever
But I wonder if I got the better deal

Jenny does it ever end, said the voice
I have no answers
But if it helps to be there I will
For as long as I can
For her voice is the voice of every mother
Of a child that has mental illness.

Lydia Chalk

Dedicated to Christian's present CPN, Lydia Chalk. Lydia is an excellent CPN.

A good nurse

How to define a good nurse is very apparent to me
Their role isn't just about nursing, as over the years I could see
Above all, they will need compassion, humility and caring
Its about putting the patient first in the closest of bonds they're sharing

Its about involving the family in their equally hard plight
Its helping them to hold onto hope, when it disappears from sight
A good nurse shows much respect; what an amazing part respect plays
She carries these attributes through 'til we begin to see better days
Its then she can reap her rewards, simply putting these qualities first
'Til at last we can see the results and define what I call a good nurse

Weymarks Way

This poem is dedicated to the staff at Weymarks. They are really good people. I know by experience how much patience is needed to deal with this illness and, as the poems explain, patience is something they are never short of. Sometimes Christian is affected by one of the other patients. I am not going into detail in this poem, as that would not be fair.

I have many memories of Christian's stay at Weymarks. He was there for two and a half years. Sometimes, especially in the beginning, he would be so confused that we'd pick him up and after ten minutes have to take him back for yet another chat with his nurse. They were very often young men, not very much older than him.

Weymarks Way

When you took your place at Weymarks
We all found it hard to cope
We tried to support each other
Preserving a little hope

Schizophrenia: A Mother's Story

You would ring almost every evening
And beg us to take you home
You sounded so isolated
So sad, so lost, so alone

You said we were wicked parents
And how much you hated it there
Far to ill to notice
How much we really did care

We tried so hard to convince you
That we would have you home if we could
We were not just uncaring parents
And that Weymarks was for your own good

You kept threatening to run away soon
And that you could not cope for much longer
We repeated time and again
That in time you'd be feeling much stronger

One thing that gave us comfort
And helped us make it through
Was the dedication at Weymarks
And the care that was given to you

An incident I remember happened a long time ago
Your nurse was going off duty
When you said, "I'm anxious you know"
You were most disturbed about something
From another patient you'd heard
She sat and quietly listened
She took in your every word

She told you "Christian, don't worry"
"What he told you just isn't true"
I started to feel more relieved
As her patience got through to you

I could see you were feeling better
I watched you become more calm
Her understanding convinced you
That he hadn't meant any harm

This was one isolated example
Of problems faced every day
Not such an unusual occurrence
Kindly handled in Weymarks way.

Thanks

The first person I'd like to thank is, of course, Christian for allowing me to publish this book. He has read parts, but it will have to be done slowly like everything else. Sometimes he says "I don't know if I really want people reading about me", but when we explain that it may help other people, he soon comes round because he knows the depth of their suffering; thanks to my family: aunts, uncles and cousins.

My immediate family, you all know about because of the dedications I've done for them individually. I'd also like to thank firstly, Colin, Christine's husband who has had so much to cope with, yet has given us 100% support always. Special thanks to Neil, Heidi, Keith and Debbie, and to Chirstian's present CPN, Lydia Chalk. Now I will write the names and a few words for them.

- ❖ Kim Forder, Christian's Social Worker—she has been excellent
- ❖ Sheila Kemp for her help and support—Alan and Sharon for being there
- ❖ Kevin Skinner/Peter Smith for their patience with my writing and for offering Christian a job, it helped no end
- ❖ Thanks to Laurie for listening
- ❖ To all my friends at work who have patiently listened over the years with special thanks to Paula, Anne and Mary and to all those that have taken time to read this book
- ❖ Special thanks to Karen Raven, Malcolm Louth, Darren Edwards (and to Celia for so much sound advice); and Maureen Allwright for her constant understanding
- ❖ Thanks to my friends whose sons also suffer from schizophrenia. They've helped me no end especially Margaret, Irene, Dave, Doreen, Julie
- ❖ Not forgetting Dr Adrienne Reveley for her understanding, compassion and advice
- ❖ Thanks to Niamh and Grainne for their help in preparing it for the publishers. And to my best friend Sherry who's been there for me ever since she found out what happened to us
- ❖ And last, but not least, thanks to my publishers for giving me the opportunity to tell our story in the hope that it might help others.

Jackie and Dave

I'd like to mention Jackie and Dave, friends of mine, as I admire them very much. Jackie had cancer when she was 18 years old. Due to this, she had a total hysterectomy, and after extensive chemotherapy lost all of her hair.

Jackie recovered and was clear for 12 years. Two years ago, she became ill again and went through the same trauma all over again. Jackie and Dave have helped me without knowing it. When I have felt unable to cope I have thought of them and the strength that they have needed to go through so much. Jackie is always cheerful and positive and I will always admire her.

Jackie and Dave got married in Southend Hospital on 27th January 2000; tragically, she lost her fight for life on Saturday 5th February 2000. She is sadly missed by all.

Although Jackie and Dave are not relevant to this part of the book, I just felt that I would like to include them, as I will always admire them both.

A letter from Karen

I felt I must add this letter. I found it both moving and enlightening. There's a lot of criticism of young people in this day and age, but this letter proves that there are intelligent and caring people out there.

Karen had her first date with her fiancé Richard in July 1995. They became engaged in January 2000. Richard was tragically killed in an accident at work on 26th January 2000, aged 22 years.

I'd like to believe that Karen was destined to read the book and I'm pleased that she feels it has helped her, if only in a small way.

Dear Georgie

Thank you for letting me read your story. It's quite strange, I don't know your Christian, but after reading your books I feel like I know him so well. It was so honestly and personally written, it really touched my heart.

When you lent me the books you said it would all be worthwhile if it only helped one person to understand about what Christian's going through. Well you have achieved that already: you made me not only understand more about this tragic illness but you also made me realise how selfish I had been lately. After loosing someone I care so dearly for, I thought I was the only person that was suffering, feeling bitter towards the world. I now feel differently after reading your story, and knowing how strong you have been. I know that every time I feel sad or angry, I will think of you and your family, and how strong you have all been through such a very difficult time.

We all suffer pain in life. I now realise that and accept it, it's a way of life, but we all get luck and happiness too, and I sincerely wish your Christian the very best of luck. How lucky he is to have such a supportive and caring family around him.

Thank you Georgie. I can't even begin to explain how much reading your book has helped me, comforted me in a way, and even made me a stronger person.

You will always be in my thoughts and prayers.

Kindest regards

Karen Raven (a friend)

Preface

Schizophrenia is a chronic, disabling disease and one of the most devastating of all illnesses, causing incalculable suffering to both patients and their families, as this book so aptly demonstrates. The poems are reflective of a journey that, unfortunately, far too many patients and their families have to make. It encapsulates the hopelessness of the situation, the frustration and, finally, the glimmer of hope.

Schizophrenia is far more common than most people realise, affecting one in every 100 people world-wide, more people than Alzheimer's disease or multiple sclerosis—people in all races, in all cultures and in all social classes. Yet the general public knows very little about it, and it is rarely publicised. Patients can, and do, improve enough to lead independent, satisfying lives—but one of the keys to this is medication appropriate to the individual's needs. Clozaril is known as the 'gold standard therapy for treatment-resistant schizophrenia', and yet it took seven years and a mother's determination and unwillingness to give up before it was prescribed for her son. As such, it is a tragic indictment of the current public health system—which works so well for some and so poorly for others.

The book is a counterbalance to the negative perception of people with schizophrenia so often portrayed in the media. Those of us, who work closely with the NHS, know that work is progressing on disseminating best practice; this story shows that it cannot afford to wait or to fail, and the policy makers and health service managers should read this book, if they are in any doubt.

Julia Bileckyj is the manager of the Clozaril Patient Monitoring Service and is a qualified member of the Institute of Healthcare Management.

Part I—A mother's story

The beginning

This is a story about the immense courage shown by my son Christian. It is also a story of hope; a 10-year-journey through mental illness, taken not only by my son, but also by his family who love him dearly. I can honestly say, hand on heart, that every word that you read is true.

It will appear from these poems that, what I call the crisis times, are the worst part of this illness, but, on reflection, I think it is the sheer relentlessness of schizophrenia that is the worst part of all. It is almost cunning the way that it lulls you into a false sense of security, only to be followed time and again by bitter disappointment when the monster decides to rear it's ugly head again.

Christian is either plagued by his thoughts, moods or feelings and this, in turn, effects, or should I say, 'infects' his loved ones. There are things that will always remain private and that I would not write about, but I cannot think of a life event that would be much harder to deal with. This illness affects the very core of the sufferer, as I said before. Thoughts, moods, feelings—in other words, the things that make us the people we are.

Two of the clients that have lived with Chris for the past 24 months (Paul and Sid) are so very kind to him. They all look after each other. When Chris goes back to Weymarks on Sunday night, they are waiting to welcome him back. Humility comes naturally to these gentle souls.

To develop this condition at any age is devastating, but I feel it is worse if you are only fifteen years old. Looking back, this is about the age that Christian started to show signs of it. To develop it so young makes recovery all the more difficult, as he had no experience of work, socialising, driving etc.

I get frustrated about the ignorance attached to mental illness. A supervisor at work asked me, "how did he catch it?", as if it were an airborne virus. In retrospect, I should have touched her arm and said "just like that". I have also been asked if my son is violent. People just assume that people with this illness are axe-wielding maniacs, probably one of the reasons why I could not say **schizophrenia** for years. All the sufferers I have met have been the gentlest souls. It's almost as if they are too good for this world. If you listen to the words of "Vincent", the singer says "This world was never made for one as beautiful as you". Vincent Van Gogh was a sufferer. I love this song as the words are very true.

Where do I start? For me this is the hardest part, as I find it much easier to write in verse. Before Chris became ill, I would write poems (mostly for my family) and always funny. I would never have dreamed that this could happen to us, but that is life. No one ever knows what the future holds and there are times when I think that is just as well.

Looking back to Christian's childhood, I can see that he always had problems, although he was the best baby you could ever wish for. He slept

1

right through the night from the day he was born. We called him smiler because he would beam all the time. As he grew older, he would be very difficult, especially after he had a haircut. My sister-in-law, who is a hairdresser, would often say that when we have our hair cut, it can sensitise us and, I suppose, as Chris was highly sensitive, it would affect him more than most people. When we took him away on holiday, he would keep on all week about going back home. Sometimes he would run away. He played up so much when we took him to Wales that I took a photo of Paul and Stephen holding him head first over a cow pat. Again, this was after he kept running away. The signs were there; we just did not see them.

When he was 15 years old, his history teacher (Mr Callow) phoned me to say that something was wrong with Chris, but he did not know what it was. He said that his concentration had become very poor and that the interest he had always shown in history was diminishing at an alarming rate. Although I was worried about it, I really thought it was just a phase that would pass, eventually.

His behaviour also changed, but very gradually; he became withdrawn, argumentative and very stroppy. He would sometimes stay away from home for days and nights on end and, when he finally came back, would offer no explanation as to where he had been.

Paul threw him out a couple of times. One time he came back again, after a few days staying God knows where, and stood in the middle of the lawn in torrential rain. For over an hour the rain was hitting the ground and bouncing back up and he just stood there, his long, dark hair stuck to his face, absolutely saturated. He just didn't seem to know what he was doing or where he was going. Sometimes, I would cry and say, "please don't make him go—he is ill". Somehow, deep down I knew, but because his dad was a rebellious teenager, we would always come to the conclusion that he was his father's son. I do not blame Paul or myself; it was such an easy mistake to make. It came on so insidiously, it was really hard to know what was happening.

When he started working at Fords, Paul said "it is the first day of your apprenticeship tomorrow, be in at a reasonable time, no later than 11.30pm. Paul was sitting up by the window when he came home at 3.30am.

He really hated Fords. He used to say "you don't see me on those buses, you don't know how I feel". Still we kept praying that he would come to his senses. Finally, after lots of time off and lots of phone calls telling packs of lies about stomach upset, flu etc., we gave in and he left.

There followed various other jobs and many more problems. When Paul got him one job at Palmers (trainee profile drawer) he had been out of work for over a year. He had no friends because he had just made up his mind one day that they were just not his type of people and he stopped seeing them. He was elated when Paul came home and said "I've got a job for you, you start Monday".

At first he absolutely excelled in his work. The two bosses could hardly believe how well he was doing. They said they had never seen anyone learn so quickly. Then after about four weeks, the cracks started to show and he would lose the plot and if they asked him to do a drawing, invariably, he would get things completely wrong. Nicky Palmer would go to see Paul and say "I really do not know what is wrong with Chris, but something is going terribly wrong somewhere".

He would sometimes stay up all night trying to work out why he couldn't get things right. One morning at 6.00am, I caught him desperately trying to get a profile drawing right, yet again. I made him a mug of tea, which he knocked over the drawing and he blamed me for it. Everything was my fault. Around this time, we found out that he believed his old mates were going to break into the Portakabin and ransack the place. He also thought they might hurt me or his dad. Paranoia was well and truly setting in.

We foolishly took him to Devon with my sister, brother-in-law and my mum. He got worse by the day. He was reading geometry books upside down, so preoccupied that he walked out in front of cars. He went and had his hair cut in the same style as Andy Mars (a work colleague). He even bought a pair of John Lennon glasses simply because Andy wore them. I think he felt that if he looked like Andy, he would also be able to act and work like him.

While on holiday, we tried to get him to agree to see a psychiatrist when we got home, but to no avail. He told us we were mad and there was absolutely nothing wrong with him at all. As you will see from the first poem "In the Beginning" this proved to be far harder that we expected.

At this point, I would like to say that, apart from a couple of isolated incidents, Christian's care under the NHS has been excellent. The staff at Weymarks are "Simply the Best". It is such a shame that 5% have let the other 95% of these dedicated people down.

I have been told that writing about life's experiences is very therapeutic. It is only now that I can see why; it has taken roughly four weeks to write all the poems, but I have been up day and night. Sometimes I would wake at 3am with the strongest compulsion to write it all down. Poor Paul was worried sick. He thought I was becoming manic. I would write on anything I could lay my hands on. My paperwork was in the dresser in my bedroom. Rather than disturb Paul, I would go in to the lounge and find old birthday cards, which enabled me to write it all down and re-copy it the next day. I loved writing during the night. It was so very peaceful and I loved the quiet. No disturbances from anything or anybody. It was the most amazing experience, as if somebody or something had taken control of my hand and was literally guiding it over the paper. Even if I had been awake for three or four hours, I would go back to bed and go straight to sleep, something I have never been able to do in my life before.

My mum has always said that the one thing she always wanted to do in her life was to write a book. She was very pleased that I was going to (I wanted to say "decided" to write one, but I did not decide to do it, I did not have a choice in the matter. I can honestly say that this has come as an utter shock to me. If anyone had said that I would write a book, I would have laughed. I've never had an urge to write, but I think that perhaps I have been driven by the strongest emotion of all—a mother's love for her child.

More than anything, I hope that this book provides an insight into a very tragic life event. When my son first became ill and I read every book I could to find out about mental illness, I scoured bookshops to find a book that had been written from a family's point of view, but to no avail. If I do manage to get it published, perhaps it will help other families who would like to know just what it is they will be facing. Maybe it will bring some comfort to people just knowing that they are not alone and that there is light at the end of their long dark tunnel.

I also hope that professional people read it and they may be helped by seeing things from an entirely different angle. It's so hard for all concerned because the nurses know what's best, but, inevitably, feelings get in the way and parents can't always carry out what's best.

I really do not want people to think that, because of all the things that happened between 1st June and 1st July 1999, i.e., meeting Dr Reveley and changing to Clozaril, I think my son will miraculously recover one day. I do not. But I do think that he will slowly improve and that he will go on to a better way of life. I am sure that I can start to help him now, whereas, for the past nine years, I feel that I have probably hindered his recovery (not consciously of course) by being too kind and too loving. All I hope is that this work may help some other families who are going through this nightmare. I pray that our story will give them the one thing that they will need the most—**Hope**.

Pride

The sadness that we've felt
Is far more than we can measure
The memories of it all
Not something we will treasure

It's been a learning process
From the beginning to "the end"
We thank God our son was blessed
With a will that would not bend

Without his strength and courage
We'd surely all be lost
He refused to let it beat him
At any price or cost

We'd like to shout it from the rooftops
Good and clear and loud
Of Christian John our son
We couldn't be more proud

A mother's story

The first poem is for all the mothers out there all over the world who have endured the same relentless pain as I have; it's also for the patients who have been let down by the system, I have been lucky in this respect, but I know of many families who have not been so lucky.

Remember Ben Silcott who climbed into a lion's den at a zoo as a cry for help? As a result, he was badly mauled. He had repeatedly asked to be taken into hospital, but no-one heard him. What a high price to pay and very ironic that he ended up in a cage.

Mental illness is the bottom of the barrel—I will never understand this as, in my view, it is the worse possible type of suffering. It's about time people tried to learn more about it and then there may be more compassion for the poor people who are affected, and their families won't feel so angry by the fact that they are all too often forgotten.

I would like to add that this poem is for the mothers who have been through far worse times than I have and I know they are out there, feeling the same as I did for years-isolated, desperate and desolate, and praying to God that things would change one day.

A mother's story

It's a story that only a mother can tell
After reading this book you will all know this well
It's a story that's filled with courage and pain
Endured by mothers time and again

They've coped for years with worry so rife
Mothers from every walk of life
So many mothers so many tears
This book is to help them with their fears

Like lambs to the slaughter they witness and watch
As their loved one receives the liquid cosh
In a bottle to save their sanity
We question what price humanity

Mothers who faithfully day and night
Pleaded for help to ease their plight
In God's name why were they not heard crying
Depleted by neglect, exhausted from trying

No one heard their pleas for help
No one considered how desperate they felt
Yet still we expect them to keep being strong
After battling so bravely for so very long

My heart goes out to one and all
Their eyes so tired from watching each fall
In an endless battle to try to stay sane
After being abandoned time and again

Yet hope has a way of shining through
God only knows how—I haven't a clue
So all you mothers please think on
Just like your child you've had to be strong

Your strength is a gift from God
The greatest of all gifts 'a mother's love'
So share with me in some well earned glory
As this poem begins "A mother's story"

The struggle

The beginning is about the struggle I had to get my GP to send a psychiatrist to see Chris who had, by now, totally lost sight of reality, so much so that if we dared suggest getting him some help he would say "what for? It's you that need the doctor, not me". My GP said that before he could intervene Chris had to get to the stage that he was a danger to either himself or somebody else. When we went to Devon, his thoughts were so muddled that he would walk out in front of cars; a couple of times Paul had to pull him back onto the pavement. At the end of the day, how dangerous must things be? It's absolutely terrifying when you see how mentally ill a person is, but there's nothing you can do to get help until, of course, something terrible happens.

During the onset of schizophrenia, Chris decided that he'd like to learn some basic office skills. This was after he'd left Fords and was about 17½ years old. He started a course in Rectory Road, Grays. While Christian was struggling to do this course, we received a phone call from his tutor to say that she could see that he had problems and that he seemed unable to concentrate on even the simplest of tasks. She said that they were in touch with an excellent psychotherapist named Jim Cook. Jim had previously been a professional football coach and had, in actual fact, coached Paul Gascoigne. Jim said that Gazza was an extremely sensitive young man and that, in his opinion, he was heading for emotional problems later in life as he didn't think that Gazza would cope with fame very well at all.

Jim Cook tried very hard to help Chris, but of course we were all unaware that he was suffering from the onset of a very serious mental illness. Consequently, things only got worse. When I paid my second visit to my GP voicing my concerns, he was horrified that Jim Cook had been trying to help Chris. He said that we'd probably made the situation ten times worse by allowing the counselling sessions, but of course we were so naive back then that we did not know what he was so concerned about. After all, we were only trying to get some help for a young man who was so very confused and distraught; again this was due to lack of any understanding on our part. We would never have consciously made matters worse. We were just desperate for some help, so any help that we were offered we were very thankful for.

While attending the classes, Chris met a lad from Tilbury who had learning difficulties. He was very keen on motorbikes and Chris decided he would like to buy a trials bike. They went to the other side of London by train and his friend drove back with Chris on the back. Every time he went out on it (after very little tuition in spite of our pleas) we'd wait for a phone call. He insisted that it helped him to think straight and when he was driving he said it blew all his troubles away. We can see now that he was trying anything that would give him some temporary relief from his ever racing mind.

Inevitably, at 9pm one Friday night, we received a phone call from Basildon Hospital to say that he'd been involved in an accident. He'd been travelling down the A128 towards Brentwood when a car pulled out of Plough Lane. Chris went over the top of the car and ended up minus his crash helmet on the other side of the road with a gash in his ankle requiring 14 stitches. The police said that it was a miracle that nothing was coming the other way. The car driver admitted liability and was charged on two counts and duly fined.

When we got to the hospital, Chris showed absolutely no emotion at all and didn't know what all the fuss was about. As we knew then how unwell he was, we were just grateful that he hadn't been badly injured or killed and had vowed never to ride the bike again. We did, in fact, feel that we'd got off lightly due to the seriousness of the ever worsening situation we were all in. A week before we were at a wedding reception and as always we rang Stephen at about 9.30pm to see if Chris was OK. Steve said, "Not really mum, he's stranded at a petrol station in South Benfleet, he's just filled his bike up with diesel and I'm on my way to pick him up" As you can imagine when he had the accident, we were by then relieved and we still feel we all got off very lightly. I can remember Paul saying on the way back from hospital, "what next?" Four weeks later we were visiting my mum when Chris finally broke down and we said "Thank God" thinking that now we'll get some help and he'll very soon be right back to normal. Little did we know that this was just "The Beginning".

Bionic man

When Chris finally broke down, he said that he'd wanted to tell us that things were going wrong for a long time, but he somehow knew that it was serious and hadn't wanted to worry us. When he was about seven years old, we bought him a bionic man and he said that was how he felt, as if he'd fallen apart, but the insight Christian gained regarding his illness, eventually, would be a saviour to him. I've been told by various nurses that it would be his saviour and of course I understand what they mean, but it must be hard when you know how much better life would be had this not happened.

The bionic man

A decade ago you told us you felt like the bionic man
Seventeen years old and falling apart, we held on tight to your hand
Season after season, till we saw you emerging at last
Fitting the pieces together, moving slowly away from the past
Little by little, piece by piece, your coming together again
Yesterday's nightmares fading away, a million tears wash away the pain
We must never, ever look back, the nightmare's too dark and too long
Your future lies on the horizon, God knows you've had to be strong
Like missing parts of a jigsaw, lost and yet carefully tended
We'll forget that it's taken a decade, the bionic man is mended

In the beginning

Slowly but surely losing your mind
Watching it happen, so very unkind
Your concentration is almost nil
But it's hard to convince the others you're ill

You worry too much, take it from me
He's a difficult teenager like I used to be
But he's been all night pacing the floor
Please listen to me, once again I implore

He filled up his bike with diesel last night
Ask his brother, he knows he's not right
There's really no need, you worry too much
Why can't you see it? he's right out of touch

He's fast losing sight of reality
Mentally unbalanced, why can't you see?
You're over reacting, you must get some rest
Speak to the doctor, that would be best

So I make an appointment for the following day
With hope replenished I silently pray

First visit to GP

I'm worried about my teenaged son
Something's going very wrong
He sleeps all day stay's up all night
Doctor tell me is this right?

He's probably suffering from his age
Going through that funny stage
Give him space keep out the way
He'll grow out of it one day

But he's verbally aggressive shouts and screams
He often has horrific dreams
Sounds familiar please don't fret
There's no need for hysterics yet

I'm home again I cry and cuss
Am I making too much fuss?
Another visit try again
Doctor he's in so much pain

Doctor please listen my son's ill
Overreacting am I still
He's losing touch why won't you see
Losing his grip on reality

Surely he needs a psychiatrist?
That's up to him I can't insist
Thank God he's sent two social workers
Now at last we'll get some answers

Mrs Wakefield your son's quite poorly
He's very thin you saw this surely
He'll see our consultant a Doctor Lowe
He'll show us just which way to go

A course of injections in his bum
And at last we'll see our long lost son
Nine years on and we're still waiting
Nine years of anticipating

The son we used to know

This next section is about the period that Chris was put on the depot injections. When we got to see Dr Lowe, he told us that he was putting Christian on a course of injections that would help him. Looking back I can see that he has never really been the same from that day to this. This is not a complaint, as we know it had to be done, but we do feel that someone should have talked to us in depth about the power of these antipsychotic drugs. For years I can see now that I really thought that he would wake one day and it would all be back to normal again.

Of course, the advice given to me by the nurses was all good, positive stuff, but I felt far too ill and desolate to go to art classes. I suppose to a lot of people it's hard to understand that my only saviour has been writing this book and they must be thinking "my God, you'd think that would be the last thing she'd want to write about or even think about. But it has helped me so much. I suppose it depends on the person and there are probably lots of people who have been distracted from their problems by doing art classes or some other hobby. I think my need has been to help other people because I know the depths of the sadness that they will be going through. Perhaps by reading our story, they won't feel quite so alone.

One of the hardest parts of all is trying to make people understand what it's like to just get on with your life. I do know that every one says it with the best intentions. Christian's CPN was always saying, "you worrying won't change the situation", "you'll make yourself ill", "take up some hobbies", "get out more".

I could go on and on. I was always very aware of all of this, but actually putting it into practice is another story. I can honestly say that there is nothing that can distract me from my son's plight. Writing is my saviour. Putting it all on to paper has helped me in a way that is impossible to explain. I've actually had people say to me "you'll make yourself ill reliving all that again", but I can't make them see that it works in reverse and, just like a huge painful boil, once it's burst you feel relief.

The son we used to know

Where is the son we used to know
This one's robotic his movements so slow
In a split second there for all to see
Then one small injection how can this be?

In the blink of an eye after being so strong
Now his feet are like lead as he drags them along
His eyes are so glazed so far away
Chris are you there? I'm tempted to say

Where is the son we used to know
Has anyone seen him—where did he go?

It's not all about Christian—you're also a wife
You really must try to get on with your life
It's become an obsession and that's bad for you
And what about Stephen? he needs you too

Will his condition improve? We really don't know
You know how it is, recovery is slow
We're all trying hard—doing our best
You're not looking well—you must try to rest

Find some new hobbies—try music or art
I can't find the interest I haven't the heart
But the mother's the link for the whole family
You must try to be strong or where will they be?

But these drugs are so powerful that isn't my son
I assure you it is, he's under there mum
The effects will wear off, but only with time
You know how it is he walks a fine line

Where is the son we used to know
Has anyone seen him where did he go?

Stand in the corner

Before we left for Sunnyside, Chris was sick outside Jim's house . Steve had lent me his car to take him for his depot. As he was on strong medication, he would shake a lot (it takes ages for people to be able to tolerate these drugs).

Chris and I sat opposite his therapist and CPN. Behind us were two male social workers, One was aged around 30 years the other was a bit older. I was completely aghast when the CPN suggested Chris drop his trousers in front of two men. Once they explained, I understood the reasons behind it, but I wish I had been pre-warned, as it would not have been such a shock.

I felt, and still feel, that he wasn't being treated with respect and dignity and people with his illness deserve a lot of respect and dignity, in fact, I would say that it is the very least that they deserve.

Stand in the corner

It happened at Sunnyside on your depot day
I could not believe what I heard someone say
In the room two males, social workers writing things down
I'm still appalled when I think of it now

Your head was shaking not yet used to the drug
I felt I should comfort you—give you a hug
"Drop your trousers and stand over there
It's injection time"—you just stand and stare

My mind is screaming this just can't be right
"Is there a problem Chris? you look so uptight
Eighteen years old and merely a lad
Your voice was faltering—you sounded so sad

"Can we go somewhere private" I hear you say
I'll never believe it until my dying day
The nurse escorted you out of the room
I felt so relieved we'd be out of there soon

As the door closed I turned around
What the hells going on here? Some courage I'd found
"We're trying to see if a decision he'll make"
I'm so angry, I physically shake

"He's been through so much why can't you see?
He deserves to be treated with dignity
She brings you back in a sad look on your face
Come on son lets get out of this place

A trip to dystonia

This poem is about one of the worst nights of our lives. A dystonic reaction is a very frightening and painful experience, both for the patient and for the people witnessing it. Dystonia is painful, physically and emotionally. I can honestly say that, before this happened, we'd never been warned that it was a possibility. I've never since been told that the odds that it may happen are extremely high and we feel very angry that no-one even thought to mention it to us and at least we would have known what was going on and had some idea of what to do.

The GP who finally came out to see our son was arrogant and rude, and showed absolutely no compassion. The first time we rang, he refused to come out even though I pleaded with him. All we could do was watch Christian whose body was contorted. He was so frightened. When he finally came, he told us to get him in our car and take him to A&E at Basildon where they would zap him. When I enquired what zap him meant, he said "They'll give him an injection which will go straight to his brain and release the dystonia. Thank God Stephen was there to hold onto him, as he kept trying to open the car door and get out.

I posted a letter and this poem to the doctor five years after it happened in the hope that I wouldn't feel so angry and hurt. All I can say is it helped. I'd decided to call the poem "A Holiday and A Nightmare", but Stephen said "there's a place in Russia called Estonia" and suggested calling it "A Trip to Dystonia"

Last night I was having a conversation with a friend of mine whose son has the same illness. I was reading this poem to her over the phone, when she suddenly said "My God, so that's what it was". She then explained that she went to see her son in Oldchurch Hospital following a suicide attempt and he was lying in a cot twisted up. She frantically called a nurse who said "oh, he's been like that for ages, don't worry he's probably putting it on". We were both horrified. Not only was she completely in the dark about what was wrong with her son, but a nurse had accused him of acting it out. In Anne Deveson's book, "Tell Me I'm Here", her experience of a dystonic reaction was very different from my friend's and mine. She took her child to hospital and said the young doctor who saw him was very kind. He said to Jonathon "that must be painful and distressing". She said those few kind words helped so much and this is really all that's needed. A small show of compassion can go such a long way. When you're faced with something as horrific as this, just a few words spoken in the right way can make an enormous difference.

My memory of that night is as vivid as ever and even though I wrote the GP a letter and sent him the poem and, of course, got a reply from him, five years on, I'm still angry.

A trip to dystonia

We'd been to Dorset I recall
A tragedy we went at all
Thirteen people, hell for you,
A terrible mistake I knew
You barely ate or slept at all
Gradually climbing up the wall
Your eyes dart round from one to another
From cousin to aunt, from father to mother

Lets go home son it's best not to stay
No mum you needed this holiday
At last we're home, what a relief
But what happened next was beyond belief
We start to unpack, you're looking so sad

"Mum do you think I'm going mad?"
"I just saw a monster out there in the hall"
No son I don't think you're mad at all
"I could see the saliva between it's teeth
I was so terrified I shook like a leaf"
The monster's your illness showing itself
But you're clearly unwell so I'll get you some help

So I rang my GP for some more medication
Hoping it wouldn't cause too much sedation
Shouldn't do said the doctor, should just calm him down
Just leave him quiet I'm sure he'll come round

I hear you calling me from your bed
Mum something's wrong with my neck and my head
Your head was grotesquely turned around
Your right foot suspended away from the ground
God what's happening to our lad
I'll ring the GP—Steve go get your dad

Another GP; he sounds harassed
Give him two Procyclidine; help at long last
Half hour later things are worse
God how I hate this evil curse

Rang my GP again at 11.30
Doctor arrives and acts quite shirty
Come on you lot get it together
It's so obvious we're at the end of our tether
Such sweet compassion still can't take it in
Can he not see the state we're in?

Get him in your car you'll need A&E
They'll zap him and that will set it free
Paul drives a bit recklessly, smokes a cigar
Christian is frantic to get out of the car
Mum he's trying to get out of the door
We're almost there Steve, can we take any more?

At last the injection, you don't make a sound
The nurse pats your bum he'll soon come around
We wait 30 minutes, the dystonia goes
Sadly and silently make our way home
We're home about one and straight to bed
Too shocked to speak so nothing is said
We must put this behind us and look to tomorrow
A trip to dystonia and too much sorrow

The word

This poem is about the difficulty I have had over the past eight years to say the word. In retrospect, I think that there are two reasons for this. One is that it has taken this long to accept the illness and, secondly, that the very sound of the word would strike fear in my heart. I wish it could be renamed as I really think it sounds so horrible. Manic depressive disorder doesn't sound nice, but I can cope with it a little better. There's a lot of ignorance attached to mental illness. I was once asked by a supervisor "how did Christian catch it?" as if it were an airborne virus. I should have taken her hand and said "just like that".

I've also been asked whether he is violent and this is even worse, as he is the most sensitive person you could ever know. I blame the newspapers for a lot of this, because they always print the wrong things. Ninety-eight percent of people with this illness are non-violent and there are more murders carried out by people who have never suffered from mental illness in their life than there ever are by people with schizophrenia. Most of the people who commit violent crimes do it out of sheer desperation; they are not responsible for their actions.

The word

Schizophrenia there it's done
Doesn't quite roll off the tongue
Eight years it stayed within my mouth
I couldn't quite manage to spit it out
A sad achievement, but there it's done
A label for my precious son

We thought naively they'd be able
Within weeks to make you stable
But sadly you sleep your young life away
Sixteen hours on average every day
Now you're timid quiet subdued
Not fiery, angry, hyper rude

My senses scream, my senses shout
For God's sake what's this all about?
Wondering endlessly what this curse is
Depot injections and psychi nurses
Mrs Wakefield try not to worry
We're doing all we can, we're sorry
You know there's not a magic pill
Now calm down or you'll both be ill
Make an appointment see your GP
This is bad for Christian, can't you see?

GP gave me Prozac and after a while
I'm flying high, I wear a smile
But we're both exhausted from the strain
We watch your struggle feel your pain
Split mind? split personality?
Get the leaflets then you'll see
Or just ask me, I've read them all
It's really not like that at all

For all the sufferers I have met
One thing strikes me I can't forget
Their sweet natures shine on through

Through all their pain and anguish too
They've a God-given gift, humility
So much more than you or me

So try to learn, don't turn away
Who knows it might be you one day

Fighting back

A glimpse of Ward 12

A glimpse of Ward 12 is about a very bad day when my son took us to Ward 12 so that Chris could have his depot increase because he was unwell. On the way home Chris said that he could see Muppets in the car and that the colours were very beautiful—a very hard time.

A glimpse of Ward 12

We've been up all night—I can see you're unwell
Jabbering on—that's how I can tell
You run on incoherently about your sad past
Slowly getting nowhere fast
Feeling exhausted—I must think this through
Must stay strong to sort it for you

I ring the centre—He's not well at all
I'll page his nurse and ask her to call
She rings about 10—"How is he?" she says
I know this will be just one of those days
"Take Chris to Ward 12 and they'll sort him out"
"Get me some help mum"—"o.k. Chris don't shout"

"Have you got transport?"
Yes, my older son
"Steve can you help us?"
"Course I can mum"

We walk through the passageways
Strange floors—they're bright blue
Two cleaners stand chattering
We walk on straight through
The nurse says "Sit there"
I'll be as quick as I can
We'll up your depot
To calm you young man

A sigh of relief as the needle goes in
So very much son for you to take in
The pain you have taken for so very long
You've not had a choice, you've had to stay strong

Still things could be worse, you don't have to stay
Shudder the thought you may have to one day

Thank God you're on lates, Steve, are you feeling alright?
"Just a bit shaken at my brother's plight"
"God he copes well mum, people don't know
I'm amazed at his courage, he's quite strong you know
I'm so proud of him mum he's much calmer now
It's a miracle he copes, I'll never know how"

I think he's grown used to it over the years
Chris go and lay down dear come on dry your tears
"Did you ring dad mum? Shall I ring him at work?"
No leave him for now, Steve, it'll only cause hurt
"Have to go now mum—I'm on 2 to10"
I say thank for your help son and we're crying again

Gritting my teeth for the fight

When Chris had to leave work yet again through ill health, he went back to the Thurrock MIND gardening project. He was working with the group on the allotments in Whitehall Lane. Sitting there brought back childhood memories, as over the other side of the allotment was 90 Kent Road where I lived from the age of seven to the age of 18 years when I left home to get married.

Paul had been crying the previous day because, before he had taken Chris to MIND, Chris had walked round the shop and bought a notebook and pen so that he could take notes about things he might need to remember. Paul had found this very sad, so consequently I wasn't feeling very good myself. It was a cold winter's morning and I had to take my mum to her doctor's. As I drove up Whitehall Lane, I could see Chris with the gardening group. Hopefully this poem will help readers understand my feelings and also they will see that, as I sat there, I came to realise that if they had found the strength to keep going, then so could I. This has happened many times, I have seen their courage with my own eyes. Inspirational stuff.

The memory that stands out most of all is the dreadful feeling of "who can I talk to?" "where can I go for some comfort?" and "what in God's name can make me feel better?" (short of a miracle) not knowing of course that what I'm doing right now (writing) would be that answer and not forgetting Clozaril. How well this drug has worked for Christian.

Gritting my teeth for the fight

I feel cold as I watch from the car
You've a woolly hat over your ears
As I watch you digging the ground
I can't possibly stop the tears
The ground is very hard
Very similar to your life

Georgina Wakefield

Acceptance so far removed
Though reality cuts like a knife
This life isn't what we've planned
In fact, nothing like it at all
Things were going so well
'Til we all hit a giant wall
We hit it with so much force
That it shattered us to the core
Left us in disbelief
Wondering what it's all for

But still you keep digging away
You work alongside the others
I think about their lives too
The affects on their fathers and mothers
They must find it as hard as we do
They share our relentless pain
They must try to work out why it's happened
Over and over again

They've advised us to join a group
Try to share our worries and fears
But we still can't believe it's true
So it's falling on very deaf ears
Can you see how it would help
Seeing so many others in pain
I shudder at the thought
As I notice it's started to rain

You're cupping a mug of tea
Leaning against your spade
You're not even aware that I'm here
Oblivious to how hard I've prayed
You're wearing your fingerless gloves
A present from Christmas last year
Why do they make me feel sad?
I brush away yet another tear

Then a sudden spark of hope
As I watch you all digging the ground
It ignites new inspiration
As I see the courage you've found
Behind the blackened clouds
Shines a tiny chink of light
I start up the car to go home
Gritting my teeth for the fight.

Carer's lament

This is about my feelings and I'm sure many carers feel the same. Hopefully, this explains the mixture of feelings that you have.

Carer's lament

Arms outstretched demand my time, my life is yours no longer mine
Need precious time to spend on me, painful shackles can't break free
Feel your anguish every day, want to run, yet know I'll stay
In desperation, ring your nurse, sick to death of evil curse
Forget that life at times is fun; can't neglect you, your my son
Feel I'm fading fast away, hold on for another day
Tangled by the plight we're in, where do I start and you begin?
Time I feel I can't afford, will we ever cut the cord?
Wake up from a fitful sleep, the first thing that I do is weep
Your muddled thoughts cause such confusion; what's reality, what's illusion?
So exhausted almost spent, need some peace, 'carer's lament'

Trees

Brittle, fragile branches waver in the breeze
They shake and bend precariously, will they ever become trees?
Some break and hit the ground, taking years and years to mend
The pain that they endure, we cannot comprehend
Some give up and die, we must learn to forgive
The sap that once was rising, destroyed their will to live
The branches good and strong survive and stick together
Striving on through life with ease regardless of the weather
They thrive in summer sun and withstand the frost that forms
Soak up the wettest rainfall, staying strong in bitter storms
Could they not support the others, in the hope that some survive?
It could make all the difference, it could keep some alive
So remember their fragility; we're not all made the same
Lend a helping hand and help them bear their pain
Support the weaker branches seen bending in the breeze
Then hopefully in time, they may turn into trees

Get it sorted

I have worked at my present company for the past 12 years and have worked for several general managers. Richard Johnson was the original manager from hell. I took his verbal abuse for five years before I found the courage to say enough is enough. One afternoon he rang me and asked was I any good at sex, as I was no good at anything else. He was well aware of my problems, as his step-daughter was a qualified CPN. He had a good understanding of mental illness, which makes his behaviour even less excusable. My life at home was extremely difficult and, as Chris wasn't sleeping very well, I was constantly tired. It was very hard to carry on as normal and yet I felt that I must try to keep life as normal as possible. At the end of the day, it was Christian's courage that finally gave me the strength to take out a grievance procedure against this manager, and justice was finally done.

Get it sorted

Richard Johnson, a most despicable man
I'll explain him to you the best that I can
Middle-aged, balding, five foot seven, with glasses
Favourite pasttime, kicking asses
Bombastic arrogant, aggressive and rude
Sly and ignorant, egotistical, crude

I'd try to call you time after time
But you were asleep though the weather was fine
Sleeping your precious young life away
Hours and hours of each new day

I knew one morning I'd taken enough
I was very tired and feeling so rough
Just too much abuse from this dreadful man
Must try to get justice, I'm sure that I can

Feeling exhausted from thinking things through
I rang the ops manager to see what to do
A grievance procedure I'd have to take
Feeling so tired the thought makes me shake

Most of the staff had stories to tell
Because Mr Johnson had made their lives hell
'Get it sorted' we'd hear him shout
I'm surprised that a man hasn't taken him out

Two of the managers came round one night
I must carry on now I've started this fight
After they leave, Paul goes for a wash
You start to heave, down the garden you rush

Your violently sick outside the shed
'Carry this through' screams a voice in my head
As I watch you so sick, I feel so sad
Your such a good person, Richard Johnson's so bad

It's not in my nature to feel so much hate
But it all went to seal this dreadful man's fate
Life's very unfair you learn over the years
You come back indoors, wiping your tears

And so I went through with it all due to you
Without knowing, you showed me what I must do

For one so young to suffer this way
Helped me deal with this problem from that very day

And so it was sorted, I saw him out
The day that he left, I felt tempted to shout
See you Mr Johnson, God pays his debts
Justice complete, now I can rest

Cigarette ends

This may sound completely mad
But cigarette ends make me sad
I see them lying in the dirt
A sad reminder of your hurt
They lie there sometimes in the rain
I swear they cause me so much pain
I pick them up to throw away
Out of sight for another day

For seven years Chris has smoked in his bedroom. He always flicks them outside of the front door and when I catch sight of them I get a very sad feeling and this poem tries to explain that.

The holiday from hell

After this holiday we finally decided we wouldn't go with Chris until he was quite a lot better. If you remember, the holiday in Devon was dreadful, so was the one in Dorset and this one turned out to be the worst of all. We went with Chris, my mum, my sister and brother-in-law to Herefordshire. I can remember stopping at the Skirred Inn on the way and having a meal in the garden. The sun was shining and everything was fine except for one thing. Chris had been complaining about his ear hurting and also said he could hear funny noises. My sister had almost called it off as she had developed a chest infection a week before we left. She was out shopping one day and had to come home because she was having difficulty breathing.

The cottage was in a very remote area and at night was pitch black. The morning after we arrived, Paul who has always bragged that he's never had an accident in 40 odd years, backed the car into a tree in the grounds and did a thousand pounds worth of damage. I'm sure it was because he, like me, could see that Christian was going to have problems. He was becoming more and more confused as time went on. We both knew we'd made a mistake, but it's hard to admit it, as you so much want things to be OK.

We went into town to look around the shops. Chris stayed with my mum. Already he wasn't sleeping and felt tired. As we walked round, I could see that Christine was having trouble breathing. The men were in a pub, so I took her over the road and they got her a brandy. But she got worse, so we drove to Neville Hall Hospital in Abergavenny. We waited while they took her for tests and the news wasn't good. Her lungs had filled with fluid and they said she would have stay in for at least a week. We have since found out that she needs a heart transplant and she's been waiting for four years. Christian got worse by the day. He tends to pick up if your worried about anything and, of course, it doesn't help his illness. The whole of the holiday then was taken up in going to the hospital. By Tuesday, we had to take Chris to the doctor's as he kept saying he couldn't stand the noise in his ears. The doctor couldn't find anything, so I can only imagine that the doctor knew what the problem was. He had asked Chris if he was on any medication.

By Wednesday, Chris told us that the colour had drained out of his sight and he was seeing everything in black and white. We knew then that we had no alternative but to go home. We had to leave Colin alone. Paul said he didn't know how he stayed there alone. Lots of other things went wrong, but they are trivial compared with Christine being so ill and Christian gradually getting worse. I think people should really think before they risk a holiday, as much as they may need one and as much as they want their loved ones to be able to enjoy themselves. Going by our holidays, we always say that we need at least another month away to get over it.

Only human beings

I write this to try to deal with my own feelings of guilt all those years that Chris was ill and existed only in a twilight world of mental confusion and sleep. I often wonder why I didn't do anything. I think it was because I was in such a state myself that it was as much as I could do to go to work and keep the home clean. Every now and then, I would write to Dr Lowe to say, 'he's not getting any better'. Looking back, I can see that we coped too well. There were lots of times that we should have insisted that he went to hospital, so I'm not blaming anyone. I feel that I should have been stronger.

Only human beings

Lost forever wasted years engulfed in a giant void
Feelings of guilt I live with for a life that weakness destroyed
Was there more we should have done, should we have shouted louder?
Is writing all this the answer, telling the world we could never be prouder?

Lost forever wasted years, I let them pass me by
I cannot find excuses, just forever why, oh why?
We took it lying down, surrendered his life to this plight
Lambs lining up for the slaughter, no guts, no protest, no fight.

Winters and summers passed by, autumn and springtimes long gone
How did we just let it happen, we should have been more strong
Will we always blame ourselves or in time will we start seeing
That guilt is non-productive and we are only human beings.

Relapse

The next two poems are about probably the very worst times of all. In retrospect I could see that Chris was slowly going downhill after my eldest son left home. After we went on holiday to Hereford in October 1997, Chris became more ill by the day. He saw everything in black and white, the colour was drained from his sight. He gradually got worse and was taken to hospital on December 27th 1997.

The week that followed was almost unbearable. We were both totally exhausted and slept until 2pm most days; we took a week off from work. Everything felt completely unreal—as if we were looking at life through a pane of glass. We had an emergency appointment with Chris's nurse the day before he was admitted to Ward 12.

We have never been able to understand the logic in her saying "you two go away for a few days and leave Chris at home". He hadn't slept for six nights. I do know that nurses try to keep situations calm, but it was so very obvious how ill he was at this stage and for the life of me I can't understand where she was coming from.

Relapse

I wasn't there when they took you in
Wanted to be, but I couldn't have been
We'd sat up smoking night after night
Just couldn't cope so I gave up the fight
The night before at A&E
A duty psychiatrist we had to see
She sat writing notes about things you were saying
Me? I just sat there silently praying
Praying they wouldn't suggest you stay in
But I knew they could see the state you were in
I recall the doctor had a very bad cold
She was Jamaican—not very old
She talked to her colleague about going away
Said she needed the rest and was going next day
It seemed so ironic as I knew the feeling
But I chose to stay quiet and stare at the ceiling
Night after night I'd been without sleep
Such a strong inclination to collapse in a heap
She asked lots of questions—referred to your notes
Blew her nose constantly and cleared her throat
As she turns the pages I can see
Lots of letters from Dr Lowe to me
I see them so clearly through my tears
They're letters I've written over the years
After much pleading, she lets you come home
Armed with two Artivan® to help you calm down
A giant mistake and still you're not well

We've prolonged the agony I can tell
Not looking forward to the next morning
Totally exhausted—constantly yawning
Emergency appointment to see your nurse
With each second that passes, things only get worse
We'll meet at the centre—be there by ten
Paul takes the day off to support us again
She's late arriving—still nothing new
You're looking quite ill and I worry for you
At last we're seated—"what's the problem?" she said
Must hold it together sort out my head
"There's really no panic, leave him alone
You two go away and leave Chris at home
You'll be fine Chris of this I'm sure"
We stare at each other, gob smacked once more
"I could stay with my auntie just for a while"
"What a great idea Chris" she gives you a smile
"Have you got 10p? is she on the phone?
Try to ring now Chris, she can only say no
You come back looking flushed, she say's it's ok.
She hasn't a clue you're in such a bad way
A phone call next morning, you'd been up all night
Pacing the floor, they knew you weren't right
Paul's getting up now I hear him cough
"I'll get him to Basildon, I can't put this off"
I don't feel I can cope Paul
"Then it's best you don't come
Who can I phone, my sister, my mum?
Paul takes over now he's really quite tough
He looks exhausted, he's, well, had enough
We've been so short-sighted, our decision was wrong
We're both feeling weak, but we must carry on
"Ring back and tell them I'll pick Christian up
Don't make me tea I'll just throw it up"
They said you resigned yourself to your inevitable plight
You remained very quiet and gave up the fight
I feel very sad now sitting at home
Never before have I felt so alone
The next week just passes, we're both off work
We've never known such unbearable hurt
We sleep endless sleep, slowly rising round two
Constantly talking and thinking of you
We've done the best thing, it's all for the best
This relapse has certainly set us a test

Ward 12, Basildon

Looking back, I can see it was the fear of the unknown with Ward 12. We met some lovely people when Chris was in there (staff and patients). If I had to go through all this again, I would certainly insist that Chris goes into hospital, as it is really the only way. I don't know how we coped for all of those years.

For anyone reading this faced with a similar situation, please try not to be scared. We found that all the support we received was very helpful. We thought that we had faced our worst fears during the seven years Chris was home. When he was admitted to Ward 12, the hurt and emotional turmoil was almost unbearable, made worse by the fact that it was two days after Christmas, which is usually a very happy time. Then came New Year's Eve when most young people are out having the time of their lives.

In retrospect, we can see that he had slowly been getting worse since Stephen left home in May of that year. We should have asked for help sooner, but Chris hated the idea of going into hospital; we have learned from all of this. The staff in Ward 12 were excellent and we are very grateful to them.

When anxiety becomes so bad, you tend to become almost numb—after our first visit to Chris on Ward 12, we went straight from the hospital to Basildon town centre to buy him some toiletries. We both felt as if we were viewing life behind a huge pane of glass. We didn't really know what we were doing. I can remember trying to step onto an escalator and it seemed ages before I was able to do so. The tiredness was also unbelievable. We were sleeping until about 2pm and, although neither of us were going to work, it seemed as much we could do to keep the bungalow tidy, in fact, even that took a great deal of effort. We lived on take-away meals, as to cook would have been too much to cope with.

Ward 12, Basildon

I've been here before, just once before
I furtively peep behind the door
One patient sits rocking, another just stares
God I'm so frightened, so very scared
What were you scared of ? I hear you say
Never dreamt that my son would be here one day

He's in that cubicle just getting dressed
At this moment he's feeling somewhat depressed
It's to be expected; it's his first stay
I've such a strong urge to take you away
It makes me feel sad as I look at your hair
It stands up on end not that you care
This isn't like you, you're usually so smart
God this is really breaking my heart

How are you Chris? I must try to be brave
I'm exhausted mum, I could do with a shave

Georgina Wakefield

Don't worry about that son, I hear your dad say
Back comes the urge to take you away
Away somewhere safe where you're free from pain
An urge we've experienced time and again
It's never been quite this strong before
I worry for Paul—can he take much more?

I feel so unreal dad—as if I don't exist
We hold both your hands and give you a kiss
Your reactions are stunted painfully slow
The nurse comes back in and says it's time to go
Stay home for a few days and get some rest
He's on strong medication
So it's all for the best
So we stay at home for a couple of days
Life passes us by in a kind of haze
We're both feeling numb it all feels unreal
I worry for Paul as he's looking quite ill

At long last the phone rings on the third day
I've been so very ill mum—I hear you say
I've just laid on my bed, paralysed stuck
I tried very hard, but I couldn't get up
I saw spiders tentacles in Jimmy's head
It all seemed so real, I thought he was dead
Jimmy's just fine Chris, he's here with me
Try to calm down, you'll get better you'll see
But they crawled through the walls, the floors and the ceiling
It was terrible mum—you don't know how I'm feeling
Just hang on in there, try your best to be strong
But what's happening mum? It's all going wrong

Benjamin

(When we went to see Chris he introduced us to another patient)
Mum this is Benjamin—he's unwell too
I'll ask him if he'll sing for you
So Benjamin sang whilst we observed
The loveliest voice we had ever heard
He sang Mary's Boy Child on this bright winter's day
With a voice that could take your breath away

['A long time ago in Bethlehem
So the Holy Bible say.......']

Patients and nurses turned around
Soaking up this beautiful sound
A perfect moment, one I'll never forget
I dare say there's more to experience yet

25

It's hard to believe it's New Year's Eve
There were no celebrations, all we do is grieve
I'll never forget it, we all shed a tear
We told ourselves things would get better next year
Can't bear to think of you over there
Such a strong urge to come and stroke your hair
You should be with young people enjoying your time
Not in a psychi ward in bed by nine

Five weeks you were in there, time went grindingly slow
We made an appointment to see Dr Lowe
We'll meet on the ward be there by three
Is Chris allowed home yet? we'll just have to see
As we enter the room, we feel the support
We're feeling exhausted emotions are fraught
Dr Lowe shakes our hands and shows us a seat
There's some people here I would like you to meet

Talks and discussions about what to do
We reach an agreement on what's best for you
A rehab centre, we've secured him a place
Yet another decision that's so hard to face
By this stage we feel at the end of life's tether
So bathed in support we'll face it together
We reluctantly accept that you're not coming home
At long last we feel that we're not quite so alone

The smoking room

When Chris was in Ward 12, we spent a lot time in the smoking room. It was long and narrow, rather like part of a corridor. Sometimes, it would be standing room only. You tend to find that most people with mental health problems can't suffer the horrendous symptoms without the comfort of a cigarette. One of the patients I will never forget is Des, who was in a manic phase while Chris was in there. He would tell us the most amazing stories. When Des is manic, he has no control over his spending; he said he's either got it all or he's got nothing. Although the stories seemed far-fetched, you instinctively knew they were true. He was one of the most entertaining people I've ever met. Manic depression had certainly been in the family genes, as both his mother and his sister had committed suicide.

Chris and Des would go on late night walks. I often imagined them together and it would comfort me. I could see them sharing a can of coke, this confused, frightened young man and this dapper, confident middle-aged man who always looked immaculate, sharing their problems in a psychiatric ward. The smoking room was the place that they shared their stories, their voices, their hallucinations, their cigarettes and, more importantly, their relentless determination to be well again.

The smoking room

I'll never forget the smoking room, there was always someone in there
Needing a shoulder to cry on, desparate for someone to care.
The ceiling was brown with smoke stains, the tubular chairs were old
The smoking room looked very tired from too many stories told
The tin ashtrays were overflowing; the air was stagnant and stale
So many anxious faces, tear-stained, pasty and pale
The grey smoke filled up the room, billowing, swirling shapes
A wog box stood in the corner, playing various tapes
Some would stare out of the window, stunned by the fact they were there
Others would wring their hands, or keep running them through their hair
I wanted to turn and run into the fresh night air
 'Til I looked at my frightened son, I had to show him I care
No, I'll never forget the smoking room; its sadness, its look and its smell
My soul will carry the memories of mental illness's hell.

Mucky Kid

There are certain things that stick out in my mind more than others. I suppose some of it depended on how I was feeling on the day. This is one of them.

We were in the cubicle in Ward 12. Paul and Steven were having a cup of tea with some of the patients. Chris was worried about his feet; they were somewhat neglected as things had got so bad after Steve left home. Chris missed him more than we had realised. We were all on the slippery relapse slope, but until things reached a head, we just carried on and then suddenly he'd relapsed and we were visiting him in hospital. I went and filled up a bowl and bathed his feet in it. The curtain went back and a nurse said 'Mrs Wakefield, you shouldn't really be doing that in there.'

I can only imagine that she could see that I was very close to tears because she smiled and said, 'Carry on now, this time. I'll turn a blind eye.'

I've included this because if any nurses read this book, they will see how such a small act of kindness can make such a big difference.

Mucky kid

You were worried about your feet, I bathed them in a bowl
I could see that they'd been neglected, it brought pain to my very soul
A nurse saw us through the curtain, I so much wanted to cry
'You're not supposed to do this, you know, but this time I'll turn a blind eye
The man in the opposite bed was rambling on and on
I clipped your overgrown toenails and decided to sing you a song

Oh you are a mucky kid.......................
One small act of kindness, but I'll never forget that nurse
She showed us much needed compassion to help with this evil curse.

True

Chris rang me one day; he'd been in Ward 12 a couple of weeks. His voice was very shaky and, at first, I didn't know it was him. He kept repeating over and over, 'I've just seen something terrible'. As he was acutely ill at that time, at first I though that he was having hallucinations. He went on to say that he'd been walking down the corridor and happened to glance into one of the wards and a young woman had just slashed her wrists. He said the blood was all over the floor. I rang to speak to the ward sister, who said, very matter-of-factly, 'Well, this is a psychiatric ward and these things do happen.' I could see afterwards how stupid it was to ring and tell her. To me and Chris, of course, it was horrific; to the staff on Ward 12, it was just part of everyday events.

True

I've just seen a terrible thing, blood was dripped all over the floor
Why on earth did I look that way? What on earth did she do that for?
You must get me out of here; it's such a depressing place
I can't get it out of my mind; the look on that young girl's face
Send Dad to get me Mum; don't leave me here tonight.'
'Calm down, try to put it behind you; it's given you quite a fright'
'Are you saying you're leaving me here? These people are so very ill'
'Please go to see your nurse; maybe she'll give you a pill'
'How on earth do you think I can cope? You don't really expect me to?'
A memory of Ward 12, and every word of it true

Why does it have to be me?

This poem is about my sister. Many times, she's talked to me about her feelings. When she realised what was wrong with Chris, she even made an appointment with her psychiatrist and she asked him what he thought was wrong with Christian. He said, 'From what you've told me, your nephew is suffering from schizophrenia'. He said he thought that we should be told and that as soon as it's obvious to him that someone is suffering from it (it is usually apparent after about two years) he tells them and their family so that they know what they are dealing with. My sister reads a lot (because her heart condition prevents her from doing much more) consequently, she reads lots of books on the subject. The more she read, the more convinced she became that her doctor was right. I've based this poem on the conversations we have had about the dilemma she found herself in. Although she knew it was the right thing to do, she couldn't bring herself to hurt us.

She says sometimes she'd think, 'I'll ring Paul at work and talk to him', but she'd back out of it when she thought about how very hard he was finding things too.

Georgina Wakefield

Why does it have to be me?

How on earth do I tell them?
And why does it have to be me
I feel it's my obligation
To tell them what I can see
I've read so many books on the subject
I've been very determined to learn
But sadly what I've discovered
Has given me cause for concern

How on earth will they accept it?
Could I if it happened to me?
How on earth do I broach the subject
Should I be trying to make them see?
Why haven't the doctors told them
It's gone on for far too long
How can they start to accept it
When they don't really know what's wrong

Why can't I find the courage
We love each other it's true
Where in God's name do I begin
When they don't seem to have a clue
Perhaps they just can't believe
It's far too painful for them to accept
So many times I've wondered
And so many times I've wept

Colin feels I should tell them
But we tend to disagree
Am I right to keep it a secret
Do you think they would have told me?
I'm talking about schizophrenia
The word that strikes fear in me
It doesn't paint a pretty picture
Should I be trying to make them see

I'm ashamed that I'm not stronger
We're so close, it's so absurd
It's right on the edge of my tongue
Yet I still keep avoiding the word
This time I'm determined to tell them
It's my duty to make them see
I don't really feel that it's fair, though
Why does it have to be me?

We lost our son

This poem describes the loss we feel as parents. You grieve for years for what your loved one used to be and you long to have a normal conversation with them. It's a very cunning illness because at times it leads you into a false sense of security. This is when they go through a good patch and you all start to relax and think things are getting better only to be followed by bitter disappointment when they go downhill yet again.

We lost our son

We lost our son, he just went away
We don't know the year, the month, or the day
He brought us such joy, such love, and such pleasure
We've so many memories of him that we treasure
We didn't notice that he'd really gone
There were no goodbyes, we just lost our son
It wasn't apparent, it crept up so sly
His dad didn't notice and neither did I.
It erupted one day, we remember so well
The very first day of his journey to hell.
He was so very vibrant, you could say a case,
To keep up with Christian was quite a fast race
Witty, lively, intelligent, bright
At 16 came the battle he was destined to fight
He's fought it so bravely through many long years
Through hallucinations, voices, confusion and fears
He stares at some photos taken of him
The tears start to flow, they fall from his chin
He tries very hard to find Christian again
We witness his anguish, we feel all his pain
He runs his long fingers through his dark hair
It's such a cruel world mum, life's so unfair
We watch his dreams shatter with every new day
The harder the fight, the harder we pray

We lost our son he just went away
We don't know the year or the month or the day
It crept up so slowly, insidiously
So sly, so cunning, I'm sure you'll agree
We grit our teeth must carry on
If it takes forever, we'll keep searching my son

The decision

Chris was due to go to a clubhouse day centre; he was taken there twice by his social worker. It seems very well-organised and we were all looking forward to Chris going there. He would read the leaflets at the weekend and we would talk about his future. He was told that some people even went to America to work if they managed to get well enough.

I wrote about the decision, when Christian's key worker/CPN told us that the Council were not willing to fund him to go to the clubhouse. We were so upset, as it was something we were all looking forward to. The manager in charge made the budget decisions and, of course, he is governed by red tape. I don't think it's his fault and I've found him very helpful in other matters.

The decision

Mr Gibson you made a decision
You made a decision one day
That the Council couldn't fund our son
He could rot his young life away
One ray of hope in all this time
Was he'd go to the clubhouse one day
But Mr Gibson you made a decision
And it's taken that hope away
Mr Gibson you don't know us
Christian Wakefield's parents you know
If Chris can't fight his battles
With us that just isn't so
He brought home the clubhouse leaflets
How futile now it all seems
But Mr Gibson you made a decision
And it's shattering our son's dreams
Mr Gibson you decide then
If our son is worth the money
He's been to hell Mr Gibson
Don't expect us to find it funny
He's been twice to see the clubhouse
We've been feeling the strain of the wait
But things have changed Mr Gibson
And it's changed Christian Wakefield's fate
Our son has never been violent
He's never asked much of his life
If you had any idea of his struggle
Of his nine years of sadness and strife
We're here for our son Mr Gibson
We are Christian Wakefield's voice
Our nightmares are still very vivid
But we really don't have a choice
That's quite a job Mr Gibson

Should be done in a certain fashion
Qualifications needed
Humanity, care and compassion
Do you have a family Mr Gibson
A son perhaps, a wife
When you make your budget decisions
You're dealing with somebody's life
Could you possibly reconsider
As to us it doesn't seem right
We're determined to make his voice heard
And we'll never give up the fight
So we implore you Mr Gibson
Try to see this from where we are
So near to some hope Mr Gibson
So near and yet so far

Another Saturday night

Saturday nights are always difficult, as most young people are out enjoying themselves and Christian is stuck in with us. He is such a smart young man and it seems such a waste to be in with his middle-aged parents.

Another Saturday night

Another Saturday night yet another one
Another Saturday night robbed of your fun
I glance over at you a good-looking lad
So smartly dressed it makes me so sad
Another Saturday night and you are stuck in with us
You always accept it you don't make a fuss
You would think I'd be used to it after nine years
But Saturday nights still reduce me to tears

As you grew older we used to say
That one will break some hearts one day
But that hasn't happened it wasn't your fate
We have tried to stay patient through such a long wait
The evil people who sail through this life
Without even a fraction of your pain and strife
But it's really quite futile to keep asking 'why me?'
We have gone over that too many times you see

So we just carry on in the hope that one day
With good medication it will all go away
You'll just swallow a pill to put things right
Then it won't be another Saturday night.

Desperate 'phone calls

Christian has been at Weymarks for 21 months now. This poem describes the desperate phone calls that we receive from Chris on a regular basis. We end up feeling sad and frustrated that we can't help him, as words are so inadequate. Bizarre as it all seems to us, to him, of course, it is very real. We can't even imagine what it must be like when it feels like everybody is plotting and talking about you. This includes TV, radio, staff, family and even people going past in cars. It is far too painful to even contemplate. You get to the stage where you are scared to answer the phone because you know that there is absolutely nothing you can do to help.

Desperate 'phone calls

Desperate phone calls and you're frantic again
You run on and you're in so much pain
You're convinced that the nurses are talking about you
I try to explain that it just isn't true
I tell you, but Chris they care for you
But hard as I try, it doesn't get through

Don't leave me here mum, let me come home
Can you hear them saying things over the phone?
Paul and Sid are as bad they do it too
How on earth can I help you to see it's not true?
Last Sunday Chris, you accused me of the same
Then why do I hear them saying my name?

I know that it's pointless when you start to cry
Listen to me mum, you know I don't lie
I'm not sleeping well, I keep pacing the floor
Please come and get me I can't take much more
Mum why's this world so cruel to me
How do I reply? Can YOU tell me?

Go and speak to the staff Chris they'll listen to you
I don't see the point mum, be honest do you?
I put the phone down knowing you're still in pain
Desperate phone calls again and again
I'll speak to your nurse who will say with a frown
Just refer him to us and put the phone down
Feel like running away with nowhere to run
It's not quite that easy when it's your son.

Sleep endless sleep

This poem describes one of the worst aspects of his illness, this endless sleep that went on for years and years. I found it so sad that Chris would sleep his life away and there was absolutely nothing I could do about it. If I called him, he would get angry. I would have to stop myself from calling him, as it would only result in a row. This was very hard to cope with, for Chris I think it was his way of coping. It was far less painful than to be awake.

Sleep endless sleep

Sleep sleep endless sleep
Sometimes too lightly, sometimes too deep
Hours and hours of every new day
In a darkened room well out of the way
Sleep endless sleep saps your precious time
It makes no difference if the weather is fine
At a time when life should be free from care
I should call you once more, but I don't think I dare
You'll only get angry and say go away
Sleep endless sleep steals another new day

You rise around five, I make you some tea
I say what a waste, you say "yes I agree"
You're ready for bed at 10pm
It seems you're ready to sleep yet again
Sleep endless sleep and I pray that tomorrow
You may get up early and stop all this sorrow
I've prayed for years though God knows why
Sometimes I question if you really try

Sleep endless sleep and I can't understand
Why you need all this sleep when you're such a young man
One day you'll wake up out of bed you will leap
Full of life no more endless sleep
Full of zest and facing a full young life
Free from fatigue sadness and strife
This is a dream in my soul I'll keep
That the day will come you won't need endless sleep.

Jumpers, jeans, trousers and shirts

This poem refers to the amount of clothes Chris buys. He spent £700 one day. He tends to do it as a form of compensation for what he suffers. Every so often he rings his brother and says "don't buy any clothes until you have been round and looked in my wardrobe first". I'm always pleased because I hate to see so much go to waste. Sometimes, even after months, the clothes still have their labels on them.

Jumpers, jeans, trousers and shirts

Jumpers, jeans, trousers and shirts
The price doesn't matter, if they help when life hurts
Wardrobes so full that they're bursting out
Why all these clothes? What is it about?

You bring some home in a big black sack
Some still have labels, haven't been on your back

You ring us from town saying I've spent some money
When we find out how much, we don't find it funny
Seven hundred in just one go
We don't ask why, as we already know
Jumpers, jeans, trousers and shirts
The price doesn't matter if they help when life hurts

Designer jeans, coloured so bright
One hundred and fifty? Are you sure that's right
Red, yellow, black, white, green and blue
Inexpensive, if they bring some comfort to you
Shirts costing £200, designer again
We wonder how long they will ease your pain
Brown leather boots that cost one fifty
The staff are concerned they will help you be thrifty
Jumpers, jeans, trousers and shirts
The price doesn't matter if they help when life hurts

Negative thoughts

This poem aims to describe the constant battle that Christian faces every day with his thoughts. On Monday nights, Paul and I are usually exhausted following Christian's weekend at home. If his thoughts become muddled (and they frequently do) we hold what I call a post-mortem and try to sort out the confusion. People will sometimes suggest that it would be easier to leave him at Weymarks, but we know how much he looks forward to coming home. It wouldn't be so bad if other patients were around the same age, but they are much older than him. He loves to go for a walk or a swim, but, sadly, none of the others are well enough to go with him.

Negative thoughts

Negative thoughts you must tirelessly change
Negative thoughts that you re-arrange
We still find it hard to believe it is true
The battle that rages inside of you
We struggle to work it out once more
Yet another post-mortem on the hour before

So mentally taxing, yet you try to explain
The utter confusion inside of your brain
We do try hard, but we can't understand
We offer small comfort and take hold of your hand
Negative thoughts—so extremely unkind
Haunting your soul and controlling your mind

You try to be positive, sometimes it's in vain
We feel so inadequate watching your pain
Never dreamt this would happen to one of our sons
We must pray they will change to the positive ones

The dream

They say we should reverse our dreams. This poem is about a dream I had about Christian. It was so vivid that for days it seemed like it had really happened; and the feeling of disappointment seemed to last for ages.

We just expect our children's lives to follow a certain pattern, and, of course we never really think that bad things could ever happen to one of our children. They only happen to other people and then, suddenly, one day everything changes and you then realise that you are also one of those other people; you hit this big brick wall and nothing is the same anymore. All the dreams that you had are shattered. The expectations of what life should be are gone.

The dream

I saw you so clearly the other night
Relaxed and confident your mood was so light
You were working at last your long held ambition
It all seemed so strange, almost like a vision
I've got a new girlfriend, you said to me
She's really great, mum, you'll like her, you'll see
We're just off to Cyprus, we've heard it's nice
My boss say's I need it so I took his advice

Do you need a lift mum? I've got my car
I said thanks son, but no, it's not very far
With that I woke up, it was only a dream
Things aren't always what they might seem.

Innocent comments

This poem is about every day conversations and how they can affect my feelings. I can be feeling OK and then one "innocent comment" can bring me down. Obviously, it is because he is not leading the life we expected for him and this poem refers to the comments made by people who don't know about my problems.

Innocent comments

Innocent comments heard time and again
Innocent comments that drive me insane
"How are your boys, both doing well?"
The older one's fine, the youngest's in hell

No, I don't really say that, though it goes through my mind
It wouldn't be fair, she's just being kind

It's natural for people to ask how you are
"Is the youngest one driving, has he got his own car?"
He's been in hospital for almost two years
I don't say that either, I'd burst into tears
Innocent comments quite normal to ask
People blind to the fact that for me it's a task

On the surface I'm fine and coping well
I cover up the hurt so no one can tell
"My John's off to Greece, flies out tomorrow
Innocent comments that cause me such sorrow
"There's a crowd of them going, a right carry on
Birds, parties, discos, if I know my John"

"My Gary's done well he's just off to uni
He's a studious lad, not quite such a looney"
I find it so painful, I wish it were you
Robbed of your youth, so sad yet so true
I say no he's not driving, he's a quiet lad
She says "Christ you're lucky, my John's quite mad"
"He works up in town, an insurance broker
Got the gift of the gab, the eternal joker"

Like an open wound that's been sprinkled with salt
No hurt is intended, It's nobody's fault
Fate dealt you a hand, we all know this well
No trips abroad, just a long trip to hell
I say I must go now, I'll see you again
She's quite unaware that I'm in this pain
Innocent comments heard time and again
Innocent comments that drive me insane.

You're Christian John Wakefield

As I have explained, last weekend was extremely hard to get through. I kept telling him who he was and that's how I came to write this poem. It covers the things that I do to get Chris through this. He gets very angry with me sometimes, as I tell him that we will never give up on him and he must never give up on himself. I do get worried that one day he will give up the fight as, ultimately, it has to come from him and, with all the will in the world, if he gives up then we are lost.

I find it amazing how hit and miss it is when dealing with the human brain. Chris is on 300mg of Clozaril daily and it's working well for him. Yet one of the patients at Weymarks is on 900mg daily and her CPN told me it is having no effect at all. He said you may as well be giving her smarties. It was the same with Chris with Ritinsurin and Olanzapine. Neither of these drugs made any difference at all to his condition. I must say, in all fairness, how understandable it is for doctors to be very reluctant to try new drugs, as they have no idea what the effects could be.

It's very hard when they try a new drug because we so much want it to work that there are times when you imagine it is working. But with Clozaril we really could see the difference. We weren't imagining it. In fact, within days Chris had improved.

You're Christian John Wakefield

You're Christian John Wakefield
That's who you are
The bravest person we know by far
Pull on your reserves Chris
For just a bit longer
Perhaps this new drug will help you get stronger

Think of poor children in cancer wards
Think of the courage they're forced to afford
Remember the Jews? They had to cope
In concentration camps, bereft of hope
You stare at me blankly, you've heard this before
I know all that mum, how many times more

You're Christian John Wakefield don't ever lose sight
I know it's hard, but still you must fight
My eyes are so tired my thoughts are a muddle
Ask dad if he'll come and give me a cuddle
I try to imagine time and again
What it must be like to be in this pain

Imagination runs riot, but try as I might
I just end up amazed at how you still fight
I'm exhausted mum, I feel so disappointed
My mind feels so muddled, my thoughts so disjointed
You're Christian John Wakefield come on dry your tears

This new drug could help Chris I repeat yet again
It works on some other parts of the brain
'Piportil' is different it effects only one
You can't just give up—you know that son
You enquire gingerly "What if it fails?"
You look very scared, your complexion pales
We'll never give up son, never say die
Come on dry your tears, it's pointless to cry

But I have heard it works for quite a few
It's in the lap of the Gods if it works for you
Thirty percent get better quite fast
Within six weeks some improvement at last
Thirty percent can take longer, could be five years
I repeat yet again, come on dry your tears

The rest of the patients? No better, no worse
But still they keep fighting this evil curse
But even for them there's much more hope
New drugs coming out to give them more scope
You rise to your feet wiping your tears
I can still get through, even after nine years
You're Christian John Wakefield, that's who you are
The bravest person we know by far.

A human being

I sent this poem to 'The Sun' newspaper and asked them why they portray people with mental health problems in such a dreadful way, often referring to them as 'sickos' 'schizos' 'psychos' and 'nutters'. The amazing part is that reports on Christian's doctor who was accused of abusing patients, refer to him respectfully. How can someone so very evil (and mentally stable) be treated with respect and yet people that are ill, through no fault of their own, have to suffer the sheer degradation of reporters who probably don't know the first thing about this subject. 'The Sun' rang me at work to see if I would object to them passing on my work to the magazine supplement of the 'News of the World'. Christian decided he didn't want to go ahead with it and as far as I am concerned that's ok. They didn't even acknowledge the point that I was trying so hard to make, which is quite typical of attitudes towards mental illness. In fact, I didn't hear any more about the article either.

A human being

A paranoid schizophrenic went berserk today
A paranoid schizophrenic is what some papers say
A paranoid schizophrenic and not a human being
So stark, so cruel, so obscene
And so hard for his family seeing
Their son portrayed in this way
Would it not be better to say
Mr so-and-so lost his mind
Desperately trying to find
A way out of this evil hell
But insanity dragged him down well
Into a lonely dark hole
How sad for this wretched soul
For years he's tried in vain
And has suffered unbearable pain
So reporters please think on
Imagine this schizo's your son
Consider the family he's had
Who know in their hearts that he's not bad
Spare just one thought for his mother
Who sadly has yet to discover

That she's lost her beloved son
And the nightmare's have only begun
Now forever destined to grieve
She'll find it so hard to believe
That the son she knew only too well
Fate has sent on a journey to hell
A tragic victim of life
Who would love a job and a wife
But the functioning of his sick brain
Forces him to remain
Locked in his mental confusion
Where normality remains an illusion
He's been sadly hit by a curse
What he got was a psychic nurse
He should never be abused
Sicko, psycho, schizo, nutter
Don't tread him further down into the gutter
But sicko's a word that speaks LOUD
Drawing in a far bigger crowd
Don't expect us to find it funny
Obscenely, it's all down to money
The tabloids get a far bigger wad
Now it's time to spare us the rod
Can't you see he's way out of control?
Unlike us he will not reach his goal
So rephrase what you have to say
I'm sure there's a kinder way
We families suffer enough
With our burden of life, it's too tough
Would they get the respect that they're due
If it tragically happened to you?

Poetry my Saviour

For years I have known that there was something I should be doing, although I didn't have a clue what the something was. Family and friends would suggest things; learning to type (this is something I wish I had done on reflection) painting, pottery and various other things, but I felt no inclination at all to do any of these things. Then a miracle came in June 1999 following my sister's prayer I discovered poetry.

It would be impossible to explain how helpful it has been to me. I'm sure that without it I would have been very ill myself by now. It is my saviour. Instead of keeping it all inside, it spills out into the paper and I feel that it is a case of better out than in. I cope so much better now and the amazing thing is that I can be awake for hours in the night yet I've got more energy now, every ounce of energy I had was taken up by the anguish of keeping it all inside.

Poetry, my Saviour

Poetry my Saviour creeping into my mind
Soothing healing gentle and kind
Quietly gently you flow from my brain
Caressing the pages like soft gentle rain

Unwittingly you provide the key
As you save me from my own insanity
You control my hand running over each page
You calm my anguish you dampen my rage

Such a powerful experience and none of it planned
Like liquid gold you drip from my hand
I wake up alert, it's 3am
The temptation too strong to resist yet again

I try to resist and stay in my bed
But over and over come words in my head
We just lost our son, he just went away
We don't know the year the month or the day

I try to ignore you but you are far too strong
The words keep on flowing they go on and on
You flow from my being and comfort my soul
My pain ebbs away as you start to unfold

I go back to bed at 4.30am
Awake and alert by 6.30 again
This time I'll not fight you
You've proved far too strong
Poetry my saviour you go on and on
You're Christian John Wakefield that's who you are
The bravest person we know by far

Paul calls from our bed asking "are you ok?"
Remember that you have to work today
I tell him don't worry and assure him I'm fine
And yes Paul of course I'm aware of the time
My faithful companion where would I be?
Without my Saviour, my poetry

I've watched you

This is a poem I wrote in 1993. I don't think I had any idea about what Christian had to face at the time. Just by reading the last two lines, you can see how very naive I was about this illness.

I've watched you

I've watched you when you felt so bad
I've watched you and I've felt so sad

Demons you've seen in the night
Never giving you respite

You've fought this battle for many years
So rarely giving into tears
A battle you have almost won
I'm very proud of you my son.

A marriage proposal

This poem describes the way Christian's emotions go up and down. It's as if he has none at all or far too many. Recently, he has rung up many times saying that he has very strong feelings for Janice or Cathy (fellow patients). A few weeks ago, he wanted to marry Janice and on Sunday night he had asked Cathy to marry him. This is hard to deal with, as he is always convinced that he is destined to marry one or the other, only to totally forget the very next day.

I wrote this poem following "Mum Do You Think I'll Ever Be Free?" The weekend was one of the most difficult that I can remember. I can see now that when he was first started on Clozaril and weaned off the Piportil, the effects were devastating at times and, at the time of writing this poem, it's obvious that his emotions were in turmoil. Now that he's recovering, he gets very embarrassed by it as he says that Janice is old enough to be his mother and he can't even understand it all.

A marriage proposal

It's Sunday night—back to Weymarks again
We're both feeling sad—you're in so much pain
The phone rings at nine, I sense that it's you
Your voice so excited "Mum I've got some good news"
"I've asked Kath to marry me and guess what, she will
Yes, I'm feeling much better—they gave me a pill
"OK I'll calm down mum, but isn't it good?
I just never dreamt that she ever would
I know she's unwell mum, but isn't it great?
We're meant for each other, it must be our fate"
"OK, I'll calm down mum, you go and tell dad
It may cheer him up, he's been looking quite sad"
I put down the phone once again you've gone high
I take a deep breath and try not to cry
I ring your brother, he says "mum it's so sad
Last month it was Janice, he had that real bad"
"Try to keep positive, Try to stay strong
He may get a bit better and might not be too long"
"Must always remember, half don't improve
But that can't be his luck mum, yes of course we'll pray too.

A holiday

I have written about this incident so I'll keep this prefix short. We have always felt guilty about going away without him because it seems so unfair that he can't have holidays. It is ironic that for most people, holidays are so relaxing and yet, if you suffer from this illness, it is the opposite. You go away thinking everything will be different and instead we all suffered so much stress. Although the cottage was lovely and the location superb, the only time I really enjoyed the holiday was when Colin drove us right into the Dales. The Lake District is awe inspiring. Both Christine and I said that we had to believe there was a God when we were in among these hills. Little did I know that within a very few years, this would be proved to me.

A holiday

We were off on our holidays, but you were too ill to come
The holiday was much needed, yet we weren't in the mood for fun
We called into the hospital to say goodbye to you
You were attending woodwork classes and your fingers were covered in glue

You looked really pleased to see us, your task was to make a snail
Your hair was very unkempt, your face was very pale
I was feeling very shaky, I glanced down at your shoes
The rings around your socks were odd, one was red, the other blue

It's strange what can make you feel sad, Sid joined us as we sat in the sun
He'd bought you a Coke and some chocolate, oh how I wanted to run
Instead I held you close, saying cheerfully 'See you next week'
We turned and got into the car, it was ages before we could speak
We must try to lift our spirits and push all this sadness away
We really must try to enjoy it; What a start to a holiday!

A perfect day

This about a day I'd sooner forget, but I also know that I never will. Chris was very unwell and had been at Weymarks for about a year in Rehab. We were sitting in the day room, which was quite full. One lady was wearing white towelling socks, a crotcheted cardigan and had a white handbag on her lap. Although she was around my age, her face was totally unlined. Chris told me that she was on 900mg of Clozaril, but sadly it wasn't working for her. An elderly lady, who'd been ill for years, was telling everyone that she was pregnant. One of the men was wearing a big overcoat and a scarf; even though it was winter, it was very warm in the day room. Paul knew I was having trouble coping. The room was very smoky and the stereo was on. At the time, a song had been made in aid of mental illness; I think it was for the charity, Mind. It was called 'Perfect Day' and of all the songs that could have come on, it was this one. To this day, I can't bear to listen to it and if it is played, I turn the radio off.

A perfect day

We were in the day room at Weymarks, a day I can't forget
The sadness I felt inside of me was by far the worst I'd known yet
The radio was blaring out 'Oh what a perfect day'
One client was wearing an overcoat, I wanted to run away

You were far too unwell to notice that there was anything wrong
Paul squeezed my hand and whispered, 'You really must try to be strong'
An old lady up in the corner, smoking for all she was worth
Called over 'Look dear, I'm pregnant. I'm so happy, can't wait for the birth'

A perfect day kept on playing; I've detested that song ever since
Made to raise funds for mental health, yet if ever I hear it, I wince
The sadness wells up inside me and I'm back in that room again
A title like 'A perfect day', ironically, causes me pain

One day son

This poem is about the constant struggle to stay positive and the conversations we have. How Chris feels so inadequate and how I try to keep him going. The problem is the more time that lapses, the harder it is becoming for him to be positive. Still, never say die.

NB: If this book does get published, at least those who read it will have a deeper understanding of mental illness. People that suffer mental illness are far less likely to receive visitors than people with physical illnesses and, ironically, they need visitors far more. Some of the people who Chris has been in hospital with never have visitors. I find this so sad.

One day son

You glance over at me I sense your pain
"One day, son" I repeat yet again
Do you know I get sick of hearing that mum
"One day son" but that day never comes
How on earth am I supposed to go on
Nearly two years in Weymarks is so very long

It's time that I started enjoying my life
Making new friends, a girlfriend, a wife
I'd love to have children, I'd make a good dad
But would they have the illness? That would be sad
Do I take the risk of passing this on?
How could I do that to my daughter or son?

I'm sick of the struggle, how many years more?
Why's this happened to me? What's it all for
My brother's so lucky, he's come so far
A job, a girlfriend, a house and a car

How does he cope? you tell me
I'm always so tired, no energy

I haven't achieved much have I mum?
Don't say such things, of course you have son
To go through so much and still remain sane
Is something we've talked about time and again
In terms of achievement, you've done so well
Still a nice person after nine years in hell

You're still very young, it's never too late
We have yet to discover what could be your fate
You'll pick up the pieces along the way
Don't say it again mum, don't say "one day"
I'm adamant and I repeat it once more
OK just tell me how many days more

One thing I am sure of that's so very true
If we tried we could never be prouder of you.

Strength

I wrote 'Strength' in 1997. It's just a short poem about the courage that Christian has. It also explains what a caring person he is. I'm sure that his illness has been worsened by the fact that he worries a lot about his family and how this has effected all of us. I wrote it when he was transferred to Weymarks from Ward 12.

Strength

I bore you my beloved son
I gave you a life to live
I nurtured you and cared for you
With all the love I could give
I fear this love is far too much
For someone as caring as you
So I must learn to let you go
So that you can learn to be you

Deep in my soul I pray
That you will recover one day
Your strength will see you through
Courage will show you the way
So remember my dearest son
Your battle is nearly won
Keep showing the strength you've always showed
As I pray God will lighten your load

Isolation

Isolation is a very sad poem in which I try to describe the isolation that this illness causes. It also explains the bitter disappointment that follows when they try a new drug and it fails to make any difference to his condition. Olanzapine (a relatively new drug had such wonderful results with many patients and yet with Christian it made absolutely no difference at all. It was the same with ritansurin. He was involved in the trials for this drug and tried it for six months, but again he showed not the slightest improvement.

The hardest part for us is that we so much want him to improve and because of this our judgement is often impaired. We'd say "He's better isn't he?" or "Can you see a difference? I can" The only time that we were certain that he was improving steadily was when he went on Clozaril. It was so quick. Within days you could see the difference and we were both sure. I can honestly say this has never really faltered. I don't think Christian began to recover from this condition until the day we tried Clozaril.

Isolation

Isolation for you, desolation for me
When dear God will we be free
An emotional roller coaster ride
We brave the journey by your side
Rising high then falling low
Spiralling down and down we go
Another drug Olanzapine
Must be patient give it time

So many times it's so amazing
We see you clearly, both guns blazing
Only to be lost again
In your world of so much pain
Maybe after all these years
Filled with heartache, sadness, tears
After struggling hard to keep on track
At last we'll see you coming back

Work

It's difficult to explain how hard Christian has tried to work over the years. You have already read about Fords and Palmers. Looking back, it was so obvious that he was ill right from the start of his working life, the very time when he needed confidence the most. Following the breakdown, he was knocked sideways by the power of the antipsychotic drugs. It took about two years for him to muster up the courage to try to work again. He managed to get an interview for a job in Grays, as a trainee dental technician. I was so desparate for him to succeed that I wrote a letter to the boss of the business telling him the truth and asking if he'd just give him a chance. Miraculously, he did. Chris had always seen his Dad work so hard and it didn't help that Steve was still living at home. When Steve passed his ONC and HNC exams at Fords, he brought the certificates home, but we had to explain that we couldn't have them framed, as we'd always said we would because it would be like rubbing salt in the wounds, when Chris had managed to get the same apprenticeship and lose it through ill health. Steve being Steve, agreed.

Chris would drag himself to work each day, totally exhausted before he even started work. During the tea break, he told me he would lay his head on the table to try to preserve enough energy to last him until dinner time. He would go to my Mum's for lunch and nine times out of ten, he would be sick on the way back to work. He managed to do about 14 weeks and only on our insistence, would he leave.

After yet another year of nothingness days and days in bed, he asked if I could ask my boss if he would give him a few hours a week. The firm agreed and gave him three afternoons a week in the offices. Just as before, the cracks began to show within about 12 weeks, but still he refused to give in. He became really run down and when I took him to the surgery, the doctor expressed his lack of surprise. He had already been told the previous week that Chris was again becoming mentally unwell. All this shows how the power of the mind operates to affect the well-being of mind and body. If one isn't working properly, neither will the other.

To Chris, this was yet another failure. I can remember him asking, 'I haven't achieved much, have I Mum?' These are the times when you want to have a good cry, but, of course, you can't. You have to stay strong, no matter if you are falling apart inside.

He didn't regain that confidence again until he went on Clozaril and this time it has been different; much easier. No more sickness, no more nights awake. This time, he went in the warehouse instead of the offices and the environment suited him better. In a week's time, he will have been working for a year and I'll always be grateful to my boss for keeping his word. There is nothing Chris likes better than telling people that he's got a job—in his own words —like everybody else.

Never ending hope

Chris has been on Clozaril for a year now and it's very obvious that this drug works well for him. The florid symptoms are much improved. They still catch him out now and then, but he gets over it very quickly and carries on with his day. He still gets very tired and his motivation needs quite a lot of improvement, but all in all, he's wonderful to what he used to be. If I get a bit despondent I just sit and read poems, like 'Mum Do You Think I'll Ever Be Free?' and I'm cured.

In 'Never Ending Hope', I've written that this condition is a curse that insists on being obeyed. If Chris wants to go out and it rears it's ugly head, it does and stops him from going. It seems to be like an emotional roller coaster ride and I wrote this poem when it was on the way down, but the downs are less down and the ups are more up. There are still times (and perhaps there always will be) when we are frightened of it coming back with a vengeance, but the more time that passes, the more our confidence rises. This new found confidence has only happened since he went on Clozaril.

Never ending hope

My pen is poised to write
I'll try my best to say
How this curse effects our lives
And feelings day to day
The hardest part of all
Is sadness by a mile
So if we appear quite cheerful
We've painted on a smile

We wonder how things might have been
If none of this were real
We wonder what you'd be like
And will time ever heal
The wounds that this has caused us
Will the memories ever fade
Of a curse that's still insisting
That it will be obeyed

Will you ever meet a girl
To share your lonely life
Will she learn to understand you
And perhaps become your wife
If anyone deserves it I'm sure you know it's you
You deserve all this and much much more
After all that you've been through

So we try to hide our feelings
And we achieve this in the main
But there are times you're all too well aware
Your illness causes pain
One year now on Clozaril
And the experts often say
It's yet to reach it's full potential
There are still dividends to pay
And so we carry on trying very hard to cope
Preserving what we need the most
"Never Ending Hope"

"Mum, do you think I'll ever be free?"

The poem is about possibly the worst weekend we've ever had. Chris asked whether Paul was really his dad. He told me I was cunning and sly. His thoughts were so disjointed that he kept saying that I'm a "Which one what" or "am I a got?" The television, the stereo and even people outside in cars were talking about him.

He rang to speak to Ash (his nurse) several times and, normally, after talking things through, he calms down, but sadly nothing seemed to work. He seems to think that, because I used to suffer from manic depression, the symptoms are the same and that's why he is forever asking me whether I used to see things. He gets angry when I say no and tells me that I just won't admit it.

The poem describes how much he relies on the staff at Weymarks for constant reassurance. When Chris is unwell, it's very hard to convince him none of it is real. To him, of course, it is very real. A very difficult weekend indeed.

Mum, do you think I'll ever be free?

You stare back at me so searchingly
Mum do you think I'll ever be free?
I'm sick of this world, can't cope with this life
Tired of the worry, isolation and strife
Do you think I'm evil? Do you think I'm good?
I can't seem to find myself, if only I could
I see dreadful things every new day
And why won't the voices go away?
Still visions appear in front of me
Mum do you think I'll ever be free?

It's as if I'm reliving such evil dreams
I repeat to myself that it's not what it seems
Yes mum I know that I must be strong
I get too many thoughts, surely that's wrong
They fight in my mind for supremacy
Mum do you think I'll ever be free
My thoughts come so fast it all feels so wrong
Then my mind's blank, the thoughts are all gone
The thoughts don't make sense like I'm a which what one

Yes I'll ring Weymarks, they'll help me mum
They help me to see that none of it's real
They're so understanding, they know how I feel
Is that you Ash? I'm not doing well
Hallucinations and voices are giving me hell
Yes of course I know that none of it's true
But how would you cope if it happened to you?
Yes I'll try harder, thanks for sorting it out
You've helped me to see what it's all about

I feel much better now Ash is so good
I knew that he'd help me I told you he would

[ten minutes later]

Turn off the TV mum, they keep on at me
They know what I'm thinking, they steal thoughts you see
Sometimes I can even pick up on theirs too
When you were ill, did this happen to you?
I'll turn off my stereo, they do it too
When you were, ill did this happen to you?
They make me confused and I can't work things out
How on earth can they tell what I'm thinking about?
Don't try to trick me I know that it's true
Why don't you admit that it happened to you?
Why do you lie mum, that's really unfair
I don't know why you pretend that you care
If you really cared then you'd own up to me
Mum do you think that I'll ever be free

It's so hard to remember who I really am
Will I find myself? Do you think that I can?
I try so hard mum, really I do
What did they say, did you hear that too?
Why do they tease me? I can't take much more
They keep me awake at night pacing the floor
I try to work out why it's happened to me
Mum do you think I'll ever be free?

You had illness mum, How did you cope?
How on earth did you manage to hang on to hope?
Nine years of my life now that's far too long
Do you think there's much longer for me to hold on?
It makes me feel dirty, disgusting and bad
It makes me feel angry, frustrated and sad
You look very tired, dad, and so does mum
Tell me the truth, Am I really your son

You're cunning though mum, so cunning and sly
Oh don't be pathetic there's no need to cry
I feel agitated, it's so hard to sit still
Why do I worry that my brother's ill?
What's that they said I'm a which one what
They either said that or I'm only a got
I'll ring Ash again, I must try to stay strong
What's happening mum, it's all gone wrong?

I'm scared that I will see spiders again
It's all so unfair to be in this pain
It's me again Ash, I'm mentally unwell
Seeing and hearing things, God it's been hell
My parents are fine, no I'm not coming back
Help me get out of this Ash, there must be a knack

Of course there's a knack Ash, there must be a key
For God's sake Ash, please tell me

You're staring again, This time pleadingly
Mum do you think I'll ever be free?
I'm stuck in it again and I can't move on
Is dad walking the dog? Am I really his son?
I'll close this one now I could go on and on
A typical weekend endured by my son
So what do you think? You tell me
Do you think my son will ever be free?

The Prayer

My sister, Christine, is one year and two weeks older than I am and to say we are close would be an understatement. Christine suffers from a very painful autoimmune disease called Lupus. Sadly, she is also waiting to go on a list at Papworth Hospital for a heart transplant, as the left hand muscle of her heart is deteriorating and a transplant is the only option. Despite all this, she is incredibly supportive. I can't remember a day that she hasn't rung me to ask how Christian is. She sends him cards to encourage him all the time.

Christine rang me to ask if Paul and I would go down to Rye in East Sussex for a day out with her and Colin. We all love Rye and go down there to stay a lot. Colin was very happy to drive so we drove over to Chelmsford and left our car over there. When we arrived, she suggested we go to Cambridge instead as she wanted me to see the stained glass windows at Kings College.

It was beautiful in there. A feeling of utter peace. Christine and I sat on a pew, Paul and Colin trailed behind as men do. A woman came over and said if we wanted to pray there was a chapel across the hall. My sister took my hand and we went into the chapel. My sister prayed aloud, not for herself, but for Christian and me. She said "God, please help Christian as he has lost so much of his young life". She also asked for some help for me, she said I need to be given strength to cope as I was not coping at all. She became very emotional and she said her voice didn't sound or feel like her own. We both cried and I said a few words for her.

To be perfectly honest I didn't think much more about it, but since all these things started to happen, I certainly have. In fact, I'd say that I'll never be the same person again. Little did I know that within one week I would be frantically writing a book.

As this story goes on, you will see that the overwhelming urge to write came to me in three distinct stages. When I stopped writing after part one I thought the book was finished and again, after part two I really believed that this was the end. Then, after a break, it all started just the same as before, flowing out words at 2, 3, 4am. I wonder why it has all come to me at such unearthly times. I can only assume it's because it's very quiet and there are absolutely no distractions. I find it amazing how I had two breaks in between, just as if I'm given a much needed break.

The Prayer—by Christine

On Tuesdays and Thursdays my phone always rings
It's my sister needing to tell me things
Sometimes her voice is loud and strong
But I always know when things are wrong
As sometimes she just can't convey
The emotional pain she's in that day

I try my best to make her tell
Of another night of fear and hell
I feel her pain right through the phone
And wish that I were nearer home
I feel so helpless far away
I'd love to give her hope and say
Chris will get better soon one day

But we both know that the road is long
Her precious son must walk along
As he continues down that road
So slow and heavy is his load
But in our hearts we both know
There's not so many miles to go
Nine years of trying to get there
Filled with courage, terror, despair

But Chris has never given in
To the torment we all know he is in
So my dearest sister don't despair
Not long now he's in Gods care
For Jesus loves the meek and mild
He'll take care of your gentle child

It's to the future we must look
So finish your story, write your book
For it's a tale that must be told
For others to read, for the truth to unfold
The journey of your aching heart
And then we'll know you've done your part

And I know that our Lord will see
You've done your bit for humanity
In his mercy he'll bring you joy
By making well your lovely boy
Another thing I'd like to say
The truth you've written will one day
Open up the hearts and minds
Of people who can be unkind

In their ignorance they will see
That this could happen to them and me

From a mother's heart your words will flow
To teach them all they need to know
Perhaps they'll stop and not walk by
For there but for the grace of God go I

Kings College Chapel one rainy day
Our lord was there he heard us pray
It's my belief he heard each word
He knew our pain he felt our hurt
And now he's with us every day
To make our sadness go away
Your son has got his life to come
I pray that we don't wait too long

The poems you are about to read mainly deal with our feelings and what it's like for us, as parents, to cope with the very hard times. Also, how hard it is to deal with problems on a day-to-day basis. I feel I'm very lucky we've managed to pull together and cope. It's very hard at times.

One day mum

This poem was the beginning of the frantic writing. I woke up and there it was in my head. I had no choice, I had to get up and start writing it down. Thank God I did. I often wonder what would have happened to me, if I hadn't started to write. I think I would have had a breakdown myself. I absolutely know that I was guided by something or somebody. It has been an incredible experience and in some ways I'll be sorry when it comes to an end.

I hope this poem helps people to understand what sadness we feel as a family. Christian has missed out on so much and the sad part is that these are usually the best years. We can only hope that, in time, he can retrieve some of the things that so many of us, myself included take for granted.

One day mum

Nine long years have been and gone
Are we any further on?
The years just seem to come and go
Recovery savagely, grindingly slow
Others outside looking in
Can't perceive the pain I'm in
They think I'm fine, they think she'll cope
I sleep, I breathe, I live in hope

I feel so sad for things you've missed
For all the girls you would have kissed
The friends, the fun you've been denied
The times I've thought of this and cried
The normal things that bring us pleasure
Far too numerous to measure
Trips abroad, parties, driving

Still in rehab always striving
Striving to be well one day
"One day mum" I'll hear you say.

When I feel I can't go on
I think of you my precious son
I feel your strength that rarely falters
I wait and wait until life alters
I never ever give up hope
There is no other way to cope

Part II—A mother's story

Christian—December 1999

I n life we learn. Even if it's about painful things, we still learn. Though this
has been hard, it has also been very enriching and I've met some very good
people; people who have been suffering for years and have not become
bitter about it. As fast as they have been pushed down, they somehow manage
to pick themselves up and carry on. This illness forces the sufferer to obey it.
By this I mean, if they try to work, stress builds up and makes them mentally
unwell again. It hampers them in every thing they do. These people deserve
the utmost respect, but, sadly, they are misunderstood. Basically, it's down to
ignorance.

One of the reasons I've written this book is because I tried to learn as
much as I could about mental illness, but there were no books available,
written from a family's point of view. I've just read a book called "Tell Me I'm
Here" by Anne Deveson and it tells the tragic story of her son Jonathan, who
committed suicide after suffering this illness for seven years. My library had to
put out a search to other libraries and in the end I had to wait for five months.
This was the only book available on schizophrenia that was written from a
family's point of view, which didn't surprise me at all.

A simple guide to understanding

I'll never understand why the mental health team workers never thought to
explain this illness in detail; it's hard enough coping with the onslaught of this
illness day to day. Even though I've read many medical books about it, such as
"Living with Schizophrenia", we always managed to convince ourselves things
would improve, or he'd grow out of it, or that he only had a very mild version
of this illness. He was different from all the others; he was more intelligent
and would be able to emerge from it one day, totally unscathed; he would
simply get up one morning and be completely back to normal. I can see now
that it was complete denial for years and years.

This poem is about our feelings after going to see Dr MacPherson, who
spoke to us very candidly about schizophrenia. I can see how, in a way, it is
very commendable that some psychiatrists will not label people, but, on the
other hand, how do you deal with something as complex and horrendous as
this when you don't really know what you're dealing with.

In 1997, I received a letter from the DSS, which stated in black and
white that Mr Christian John Wakefield suffers from 'PARANOID
SCHIZOPHRENIA'. I can remember dropping the letter crying. I made
numerous 'phone calls, one of which was to my GP who said "Well, he's on
disability allowance, it's obvious that this is true". Yet no-one ever told us!

Paul and I went to our GP the following day and this is how he
explained it to us. Call it an idiot's guide if you like but it worked starkly and

immediately. He drew this diagram. He said to visualise it like a game of battleships and that M is for Mother, B – Brother, W – Work, S – Socialising and F – Father.

S		M
	W	
B		F

He said a normal brain is able to channel the thoughts of the subject (for example) correctly, but a person with schizophrenia is not able to do this, as one of the symptoms is a thought pattern disorder. Therefore, the brain will often flit from one subject to another, making it almost impossible to concentrate and this explains why many people cannot work or study. It explained very graphically to us just why he had never been able to hold down a job for very long.

Paul then said to the doctor "so basically, you're writing my son off at the age of 24"? Dr Macpherson replied "I'm not writing him off, but, needless to say, his life and your lives will be difficult" It was only then that we started to take in the seriousness of the situation that we were in. I hope this section of the book might simplify a very complex condition and help families to understand it a bit better (as we did).

I tend to liken it to reading an instruction manual; say a mobile phone, a VCR or computer or, alternatively, to someone physically showing you how to use one of them. This very simple diagram helped us both to imagine if you like, what it must be like from the sufferers point of view. We both feel that if someone had taken the time to explain it in this very simple way years before, it would have given us a much better understanding and we would have been able to help our son more because of it. Lets face it, the carers are always there for their children; we don't get any breaks from it and even if we do manage a holiday(feeling guilty for doing so), we take it all along with us as extra baggage.

I've tried many times to analyse all this writing. I do feel that, for me, it's a very positive way of being in some sort of control of a very bad situation that you can do absolutely nothing about. I'm a very organised person and I also think that this may be the reason why this book is mostly in the form of poetry. For me, it's tidier somehow.

United

The day that the GP explained things to us simply and yet graphically, inspired me to write the next poem, one that goes on to explain what we did and, hopefully, how we both felt immediately after leaving the doctor's surgery. It's called 'United'. I've always said that it's only Paul and I who really know the pain that this illness causes. I hope the reader understands this. After seeing the doctor, Paul stopped the car in Bridge Road, opposite the park. We both needed a little time to take in the seriousness of our situation.

I remember several times when we've driven out into the countryside and just sat staring into space in utter disbelief, but at least we had each other. I can't even contemplate going through something like this without having the comfort that there is one other person on this earth that totally understands what it is like to be in this pain.

I'm sure readers must have thought what a very depressing story this is, but I can only tell it how it is. Everything you've read is the truth and there is no way to paint a pretty picture and I wish more than anything that I'd never written this book because then none of this would have happened. On a happier note, as you've read, we feel that Chris has recovered more in the past year on "Clozaril" than all the years before on "Piportil". I've read that there is a small percentage of patients who don't respond to any drugs that are available. They are treatment resistant, and Paul and I often say that this is something we can't even think about as it's just beyond comprehension.

United

We're sitting outside the park
Both staring in disbelief
United in our plight
United in our grief
But he's only twenty-four
This is far too hard to take
The son that we've both nurtured
There must be some mistake
We cling to one another
As sadness overflows
I know exactly how he's feeling
Only he and I could know
The depth of so much sorrow
The core within the pain
When hope eludes us both
Time and time again
At least it's brought us close together
Not driven us apart
This love we share for Christian
We both feel from the heart
I can feel his body shaking

Tears for his long lost son
I tell him to keep fighting
In this war that must be won
Sometimes he is the strongest
Just depends upon the day
His turn to lift my spirits
Keep negativity at bay
What would I do without him
The times I've wondered this
I wipe away his tears
He repays me with a kiss
Amidst the sadness, I take comfort
In knowing till the end
That my husband, Christian's father
Will always be my friend

The Bean Crier

On June 20th, during the night, I was writing that I will have to prefix each poem with an explanation and then it would be easier for people to understand. I would do this on a separate piece of paper and it would be easier to follow.

I heard the loft ladder creaking and Christian came down. He was drinking Sunny Delight from the fridge. He asked why I was still up and I lied to him. I said, "I was thirsty, like you."

I'd put the paper and pen under the armchair and he didn't have any idea that I was writing this book.

Chris said it was a dream that woke him up. "I was in a classroom with my English teacher and there was a CPN in the room."

He said "I was reading book called the Bean Crier. My English teacher said, 'Christian, you must read the first page before each paragraph as it will make the story easier to understand' and the CPN said 'Christian, your mum will write about the spiders you have seen'. He was dreaming of what I was writing at exactly the same time I was writing it.

There have been times in the past when Christian and I have connected in the same way. I often wonder if, because his brain doesn't work in the same way as other peoples, it is far more sensitive in other areas and he is able to pick up on things as we are not able to do. For example, one evening, about 7p.m, the 'phone rang. It was a friend from work and Chris told me who it was before I'd even answered the telephone. If this lady rang me regularly, I could understand it, but she hadn't rung me in years.

Paul's Birthday/Father's Day

I was feeling a bit strange on this Sunday morning, probably because I was still feeling shocked that Christian had been dreaming of what I had been writing (at the exact time that I was writing it) the night before. I'd also been writing that I must mention Tanya's wedding and the fact that we couldn't attend, as I was feeling too ill due to Christian being very unsettled at Weymarks, and the stress that we were under at this time.

As Paul, Christian and I were walking around Battlesbridge Mills (something we often do on a Sunday) I felt someone tapping me on the shoulder, I turned around and it was Tanya, who I hadn't seen since she left work a year before. She was with her husband, and her dad who Paul had worked with years before and had not seen in years. On the way home we followed for miles a grey Ford Orion (old type). The number plates included the letters TLC, Christian said to me "look mum, TLC, tender loving care". The car indicated right and pulled in at the caretakers house to William Edwards School, Christian's old secondary school where his dream the night before had taken place. It was at this stage that I knew my sister's prayer had been heard and there was more to come.

Christian's cousin, Heidi, wrote this poem for him and I thought it would be nice to include it for her.

My cousin—by Heidi

My cousin has an illness
The illness attacks his mind
Voices and noises in his head
It's really so unkind
Sometimes they're with him day and night
And to overcome them he must fight
He controls his thoughts to keep them at bay
Please God they will be gone one day
'Til that day comes, Chris won't give in
There's an angel watching over him

Your Shout

I get so angry if I watch "Your shout"
To hear them bleating on about
Schools overcrowded, BR's no good
Holes in the road and saving our woods
They moan about the pain life brings
Politics, shops and trivial things
There's starving babies on TV
It's all so petty, can't they see?
Can they not see, they've got their wealth
If they enjoy the best of health
If life hadn't dealt me so much pain

Would I have ended up the same
Must stop myself from screaming out
It's best that I don't watch "Your Shout"

Christian's psychiatrist said that the following incident was a very strong factor in triggering his illness.

When Chris was 16 years of age, he was on a train between Upminster and Romford with his friend Zack Cox. He'd been to Ski West and bought £200 worth of sports gear. In their carriage was a man aged about 24 years, who produced a knife and told them that he was going to kill them both. He said he would kill Zack first and when Christian asked him why he said "Because I don't like his F...... face"

He made off with Christian's new gear and also Zack's. When he came home he was shaking from head to foot. He just couldn't believe that someone could do that. The following Saturday we gave him some more money and Stephen took him back to Romford. At 3pm Steve rang me and said "my brother's gone mad mum, he thinks he's seen the man that mugged him amongst all the crowds in Romford." In actual fact he had. Christian had given the police a very good description of the man and when he went back to change the clothes in Ski West they held him in the shop until the police arrived. The police said he was a drug addict and he had only been let out of prison that very morning at 11am.

I have always felt that this was the trigger as far as Chris was concerned as he was never the same after that incident. Psychiatrists can draw their own conclusions, but it's what I feel as a mother. The shock was far too much for him. Six months later he was working with his dad during the holidays and he caught his finger in a hydraulic press. His finger literally burst open. He had 18 stitches, 2 breaks, and a dislocation. He was in hospital for two weeks on an antibiotic drip as they were worried about bone infection.

About one year after that he was driving down the A128 on a small motorbike when a car pulled out of Plough Lane, Bulphan, and Chris went over the top of the car. He had 14 stitches in his leg and about two weeks later he actually had a mental breakdown. During the year leading up to this I went to my GP several times as I could see that he was mentally breaking down.

Even though this book provides an insight into the devastating effects of this condition, I really don't think it's possible to put into words how very hard it is to deal with. How do you explain what it is like to watch your son sobbing with sheer frustration when he's been prevented from doing the things in life that we all take for granted. We often say that it's even harder than being physically disabled, as it spoils every aspect of the patient's life, holidays, working, driving, socialising and, in our son's case, even eating because he is often physically sick.

There are times when I wish he would just accept how hard it is to work with this disability, but I know he never will. Tiredness plays a big part too. The anti-psychotic drugs do have a very sedative effect. In fact, I know someone who took 100mg of Clozaril by mistake and he went into a coma for 12 hours. He says he knew what was going on around him, but he couldn't move or speak until the effects wore off. Chris finds it very hard to understand how other people can work all week. He tends to compare himself with others and ends up very confused. I suppose after ten years on these drugs, coupled with the tiredness caused by having an overactive brain, you can't even remember what it is like to have normal energy levels.

Sometimes, inevitably, there are things that can make you smile and I'm sure you're feeling relieved after so much sadness. There are quite a few things I could write about, but most of them don't really seem appropriate. This incident sticks out in my mind more than any of the others. When Chris was at Weymarks, he went out one evening with a fellow patient who was around the same age as him. They went out for a drink in town. They got talking to two girls and in Christian's words, "Suddenly I wanted the ground to open up when Richard said, "allow me to introduce us, I'm Richard and this is Christian and we're both paranoid schizophrenics" to which, one of them said "paranoid what?"" I know it must have been hard for Chris, but I had to say what I felt and that was, 10 out of 10 for guts. Richard had well and truly got past the stage of hiding it or being like Chris, totally embarrassed by it. When Chris said to Richard "God, how could you, they think we're a pair of nutters?" he replied "that's their problem perhaps they should take the time to learn a bit more about it. I can remember thinking, he must have gone through so much to reach that stage. I suppose personality plays a big part. I really don't think Chris will ever be able to say things like that. He would never have that much confidence.

Dr Reveley and the seminar

Paul and I went to the much awaited seminar (and now in retrospect thank God we did). Dr Reveley from the Maudsley Hospital conducted the seminar. This woman projects care and compassion, and Paul and I actually felt it.

During the break I called her and told her about Christian. Her first question "Have they tried Clozaril?" When I replied, "No" she said, "go back and ask for a second opinion." I said I had asked for one two years before and my GP refused. She told me he had no right to refuse. She also said that she doubted very much whether we would get to see her, as Christian would probably be offered Clozaril when we asked for the referral. She gave me her direct line number (a privilege I've never had before) I have written and spoken to her since to keep her in touch with what's going on. Ever since I met Dr Reveley, she has restored my faith in human nature. She is not just a doctor, she is a humanitarian.

Paul and I went to see Ian Beatty (Weymarks) as Paul was very worried about me. I'd been up all hours of the night writing and Paul thought, as did lots of other people, that I was becoming ill, made worse by the fact that I suffered from manic depression most of my adult life. My illness burned itself out when I past 40 years of age, and Christian's started not long after. Ian Beatty was most helpful and he assured Paul that I wasn't ill and, in actual fact, it was probably helping me to get all of this down on paper and out of my system. Paul was then able (for the first time) to listen to most of my poems.

As green as grass

The conversation between Dr Reveley and myself on July 1st 1999 (see *Dr Reveley and the seminar*) was an eyeopener. Her first question was "have they tried Clozaril?" to which I relied "No doctor". She then said it was the best drug for this condition if it works for you. She said to go back and ask for a trial for Chris. I said "but surely they must know it wouldn't work for him, and she said "how can they possibly know without trying it"? Dr Reveley said "If your son had a brain tumour, they wouldn't refuse you a second opinion". It just shows how green we were; we had just accepted what my GP had said and had gone home and forgotten it. This makes me feel as if I didn't do enough, but at the time I was very weak myself. But I will always wonder, was there more we could have done had we have been stronger. It has taught me a major lesson and that is to find out about your rights. Don't just accept what you are told; don't be intimidated just because you feel that these people know best.

I vividly remember Paul and I talking and saying even though other people had told us how good Clozaril is that it was obvious (especially as Chris was so young) they would try it. We really thought that the doctors felt it wouldn't work for him; talk about 'as green as grass'.

Dr Dean

After this conversation with Dr Reveley, we got an appointment with Christian's consultant. I went to see Dr Dean on August 10th at 9.30am at Basildon Hospital, Ward 12. When we got there, Dr Dean wasn't there so his registrar, Dr Akomolafe rang him and we could hear the conversation. (When we went to the seminar on 1st July, I called Dr Reveley over and told her that I wasn't happy with Christian's progress. She asked me if he had been tried on Clozaril. She asked his consultant for a referral. But I doubt if you will get to see me, he will probably offer to put him on Clozaril. This is what usually happened. We told his nurse that we were thinking of asking Dr Dean for a referral. Dr Akomolafe said "yes I'll explain to Mr and Mrs Wakefield all about Clozaril". He then apologised for Dr Dean's absence and said that his secretary had forgotten to enter our appointment in his book.

Dr Akomolafe then took us into a private room and explained Clozaril to us in detail. He said we had one week to think about it and Dr Dean would see us at Weymarks on Wednesday 18 August at 3pm. He said that, in the meantime, he would go to Weymarks and go through Christian's notes, and when Christian comes home for the weekend, we could begin to prepare him for a medication change. We said that we would be happy to.

Stephen took time off work to come with us on Wednesday 18th. In the meantime, Christian's keyworker, who we had told about the possibility of Christian being put on Clozaril, told us the good news was that Chris could still take his place at Kit-Kats, even if he went on Clozaril.

When we got to Weymarks (2.50pm Wednesday 18th) Chris was already in with Dr Dean. When he came out at 3.05pm he was very angry. He said Dr Dean had told him off and had no intention of trying Clozaril. He said that Dr Dean had said he doesn't try hard enough, yet Ash, his keyworker had told him only the week before that they were very pleased with him and that he had completed his care plan successfully. When we went in to Dr Dean, also in the room was a CPN and a social worker. He started talking about Chris not trying hard enough. I told him that I've seen Christian going through so much that I could not agree with that. I showed him a diary entry written four years before, which I had kept (Jan 1st 1995).

I then said that we had made a decision about Clozaril and Christian was happy to give it a try. He didn't seem to know what we were talking about. He said he had no intention of trying Clozaril. We were stunned and just looked at each other. We explained what Dr Akomolafe had said (take a week to think about it) and he did not know what we were talking about. I showed him a note from my son to Dr Lowe (written Jan 1st 1995) and said "does this sound like someone who does not want to get well?" and then he said "I am willing to try another "A" typical (ami sulpheride). Chris would be on it for six months and if he had not improved, we had his word that he would try Clozaril.

We decided to go along with this, as we were grateful for any medication change, but we felt disappointed as all our hopes had been pinned on Clozaril.

Then the following Tuesday came the Cook Report "Doctors From Hell". I cannot tell you how distressed we felt. We were both physically sick and lost a lot of sleep over it. A help line for relatives and patients was set up and I was given an appointment for 3pm Wednesday 25th August.

Stephen came with me to see Brandon Hayes. I felt very sorry for Brandon as he had to do all the clearing up and take all the aggravation caused by Dr Dean. I explained that I wasn't there because I had any concern that Dr Dean had done anything untoward to my son, but I was concerned that when he saw him on Wednesday 18th August, he did not seem to know what we were talking about, even after he'd promised to put him on Clozaril if, after we'd discussed it for a week, we still wanted a trial.

The outcome is that Christian is going on a trial for Clozaril very soon. So in a way, this sad event has worked in our favour. Now it is all in the lap of the Gods. I have insisted on a letter of apology to Christian as he was very distressed by all this, I feel that it was the very least that they could do. And, of course as the story goes on you will see that this drug has had wonderful results. In fact, we could see a difference within days.

My final conclusion this story is that there are three reasons for my son's recovery. Firstly, I believe and will always believe that on June 3rd 1999 at King's College Chapel, Cambridge, someone heard my sister pray. Secondly, Christian has a lot of courage and an iron will. Lastly, because I am so much better, I can help Christian. Before I started writing, I am sure I caused him a lot of anguish and he would worry about me worrying about him, which, of course, had an extremely detrimental affect on his condition. I know Chris still has a long way to go, but I am sure he will go on now to a far better and more constructive life.

As you read this story, you will see that I wrote to "The Sun" newspaper. I find it very hard to believe that they have the audacity to call people who suffer from mental illness "sickos, psychos, schizos, nutters" and yet, in the newspaper report on Dr Dean, he is given respect and referred to as a doctor. As far as I am concerned, he doesn't deserve any respect. He was not mentally ill, just as this poem says "pure evil".

As you will see, we were given an appointment with Doctor Payne (who was standing in for Dr Dean) at 3pm Wednesday September 15th. He patiently listened to our story and agreed to put Chris on Clozaril on Monday 20th September 1999, and we feel that this is where the story changes and it was when our son actually did begin to recover.

I spoke to Gary Wong today (8th October 1999). They have gradually increased the Clozaril from 3 x 12.5mg daily to 3 x 50mg daily. Gary said they keep increasing the dosage until they have reached the optimum level. This can be up to 900mg daily, but he said most patients settle at around 250–300mg daily (fingers crossed). His blood pressure has been rising and he has had palpitations a few times, but, even so, it is a case of so far, so good. By 14th October 1999, the Clozaril dose is 4 x 25mg daily and blood tests are fine.

A wolf in sheep's clothing

This poem explains how we felt seeing Dr Dean on TV. So many emotions. The worst part was the betrayal we felt that this wasn't a nurse or a GP. He was in the ultimate position of trust and he abused it. So many people were effected by this man's actions. We still find it hard to believe. But this was not as bad as the effect it had on our son. Due to the nature of his illness, and the fact that he went to woodwork classes, etc., everyone was talking about Dr Dean. Christian kept thinking that they were talking about him. He rang several times saying that the police were after him. It was very hard to pacify him and very sad that it had affected him in this way. There was only one person to blame and that was Dr Dean. I think what made it worse was that I liked the man. I can remember him asking Chris if there was anything about Weymarks that he would like to change. To which Chris replied " I wish that the others were around my age". To which Dr Dean replied " Oh, we've got all that in hand, we're giving all the others an injection tonight and by this time tomorrow, they will all be 24 just like you". I found this most unusual because most senior consultants are quite detached and rarely amusing, he seemed a charming man, on the surface of course.

A wolf in sheep's clothing

It's Christian's psychiatrist, Dr Dean
Pursued by reporters and a camera team
But he's a senior consultant and a gentleman too
There's been a mistake—no way is it true

I stare at the screen—I don't understand
He was so professional and such a kind man
We sat in his office only last week
We're feeling so shocked and we struggle to speak

We trusted this man—he helped with our fears
He's been Christian's consultant for almost two years
He'd exploit his patients for his own relief
I feel sad and confused, it's beyond belief

Such vulnerable people, how on earth can this be
He's as bad as a paedophile, I'm sure you agree
To prey on such people is just pure evil
Disguised as a doctor, but surely the devil
Two months have passed since this bitter pill
How on earth could this happen to people so ill?
A predator, on his patients he preys
But they'd say "she's a nutter"
"Don't believe what she says"
Unbelievably cunning, it's hard to conceive
If they spilled the beans who would believe
To use these poor souls for self-gratification
And rely on others to provide explanations
My heart goes out to his staff, left behind
He's just left them to it, how extremely unkind
They must face many families and try to explain
Families already in too much pain
They help build our confidence, as this is a must
As we're left to wonder who do we trust?

Clozaril

This poem describes what a big decision it was to suggest that Chris changed his medication. At the end of the day only he could make that decision. We are very proud of him because ever since he experienced a dystonic reaction five years ago, he has been terrified that it could happen again, which is very understandable (see *Trip to dystonia*).

Clozaril

We've heard many times that Clozaril is best
Unaware of the fact that it may be quite a test
The upside's you'll improve—it could be quite fast
The downside's a relapse we both look aghast
What do we do which way should we go
A hard decision and how will we know
Will it help you get better or will you get worse
Will it help to alleviate this evil curse
If you agree to a trial at Weymarks you'll stay

As it has to be monitored every day
Should we try to forget it and just carry on
Which decision is right and which one is wrong
Find the courage to gamble this time
To waste any more years would just be a crime
So think hard my son and try to stay strong
Might not be much longer for you to hold on

Remember we're here, willing you through
All that we ask is what's best for you
You deserve this chance so give it a try
It's so sad at weekends hearing you cry
Show us your courage as you've done all these years
Then maybe we'll see an end to your fears

Courage

When Dr Payne agreed to try Chris on Clozaril, we were ecstatic. Even though we knew it might not work, there was always the chance that it would and we desperately needed that glimmer of hope. Leading up to the Clozaril trial, he had been very unwell (see "Mum, Do You Think I'll Ever Be Free?") and various others. He was physically very sick, but now, in retrospect, it was just as well, because he was so very sick of being ill, I think he would have agreed to almost anything. Nevertheless, it took a lot of courage and he is very frightened ever since he had a dystonic reaction (see, A Trip To Dystonia). I really do not know if I would have been brave enough; still that is all in the past now and we must look to the future with hope renewed.

Courage

You found the courage dug down deep
From a bitter harvest will you reap
Your just rewards for staying strong
A miracle you carried on

Your iron will just would not bend
We knew you'd do it in the end
Determination shining through
Provides a better life for you

The courage needed so immense
We witnessed feelings oh, so tense
We'd have understood you saying no
But if you had where would you go

Just plodding on with half a life
The very thought cuts like a knife
How could we doubt you—should have known
Such courage you have always shown

We'll keep on praying all goes well
No risk of going back to hell
I'm sure you know how hard we'll pray
Until at last we see the day

You're free at last from all your pain
Our prayers will not have been in vain
Years of suffering in the past
And courage will have won at last

Questions and determination

This poem describes our present situation. So many questions, wondering if he will emerge from all this pain and, if he does, what will he be like, or if the change of medication will make a difference at all? Will he make some friends? Will he have any relationships? So many questions.

Questions and determination

Where will you live? where will you go?
Canvey or Basildon, when will we know?

Next week a new drug, a Clozaril trial
There could be some side effects, at least for a while

We all feel excited and yet frightened too
Slightly nearer to knowing if it works for you

We've read all the leaflets Time and again
Wondered endlessly, will this ease your pain

It has good results or so we've heard
Will it set free your spirit, as free as a bird

We are willing you on son, we must see this through
To discover if life could get better for you

One thing I'm sure of deep down in my soul
We will never give up until you've reached your goal

If Clozaril should fail, all is not lost
We must carry on, whatever the cost

And so we wait patiently, after many long years
Will a new drug help to alleviate your fears?

Will you go back to college, will you retrieve your life,
Will you make some new friends, a girlfriend, a wife?

Will you learn to drive again, perhaps go away?
Maybe you'll manage a holiday

Without being ill and enjoying your time
Is it possible you're at the end of the line?

Can you imagine the demons are gone
Along with the voices you've heard for so long
So many questions to be answered my son
If it takes forever, we'll just carry on

We saw you this weekend

How can you explain last weekend? It is almost impossible. We call it "a miracle". In our wildest dreams we could never have prepared for this. If we had won the lottery, it could not have come even close to the feeling of elation at seeing Chris so relaxed. I am not saying it was all plain sailing, but the confusion lifted so quickly. For years we have said how lovely it would be to hold a conversation with our son and we did. It was a very strange experience. If it felt like that to us, it is hard to imagine what it was like for Christian. We went to see him after three days on Clozaril and we were already able to see a change taking place. Like watching a caterpillar changing into a butterfly. Slow but sure, all we can do now is pray that things continue to improve. So far so good.

We saw you this weekend

We saw you this weekend, looking so well
Right here with us and no longer in hell
We saw you this weekend, making decisions
Much more relaxed and free from visions

We saw you smiling, we heard you speak
Strong and forthright, not confused or weak
Just two weeks on Clozaril, so hard to take in
The battle still rages, but so far you win

You were not just a figment of imagination
Dare we say it's due to the new medication
We saw you this weekend, so plain to see
Glimpses of your personality

You were free from stress and causing no trouble
We knew you were there, beneath all the rubble
It took the Clozaril to help dig you out
Welcome back son, we were tempted to shout

But we resisted temptation and saw some sense
That would only be tempting providence
You bought an alarm clock, which you set for eight-thirty
You got yourself up without acting shirty

On Sunday morning, up and dressed by nine
For the first time in years, enjoying your time
We went down to the beach to walk the dog
You said it felt like you had come through a fog

You were quite ecstatic, in a bit of a whirl
Coming to terms with a less hostile world
At times overwhelmed and close to tears
Amazed and relieved after so many years

We saw you this weekend making choices
Much more focussed and free from the voices
Where have I been, Mum? It all feels so odd
None of that matters now, let's just thank God

This is good medication Mum, take it from me
It's tuned in my brain to the right frequency
I'm coming through the maze, in fact, I feel fine
That's great son, but remember—one day at a time

Let's all say a prayer this will just carry on
Has the nightmare ended, are the demons gone?
We saw you this weekend, Dad, Steve and me
Has Clozaril set your spirit free?

The journey

We are really in quite a state of shock because each time we see Chris now, he seems even better than the time before. I suppose the only people who can really appreciate this book are the families going through the same thing. The thing that worries me more than anything is that there are people out there who are not getting the best medication due to money. Mental illness is a very difficult thing to cope with and, sadly, some people, through various reasons, either abandon their loved one or just give up the fight. In all honesty, I can understand this. I have been blessed with a good husband and a very supportive family. Others are not so fortunate, and I can't honestly say, hand on heart, that I would have coped without the support that I have had.

When Chris was about 20 years of age, he sat up one night and watched a play about a lady with motor neuron disease. The next day I found a scrap of paper and he had written on it "Our greatest glory is not in never falling, but in rising every time we fall". I can remember him saying "This is what I have to do all the time", and I refer to this in "The Journey"

In one part it says, "like a helpless baby expelled from the womb, screaming for comfort in a well locked room". This is to help you understand that this is what it felt like. I felt there was nothing I could do to ease his terrible suffering. No way I could reach him.

The journey

Our son went on a journey nine long years ago
Almost like eternity it passed very slow
How hard that journey, words can't explain
To know he was out there, in so much pain
Like a helpless baby expelled from the womb
Screaming for comfort in a well locked room
All we could do was wait patiently
And wonder endlessly would we ever see
Our son return safe and well
Coping with life after nine years of hell

Through a barren desert cracked from the heat
Not willing to ever admit defeat
A precarious journey filled with pain
He stumbled and fell time and again
Only to rise to his feet once more
At last came a miracle, he walked through the door
He stands before us in far less pain
Whilst we pray he won't take that journey again

Lost and found

After six days on Clozaril, the difference is incredible. There have been some problems, but nowhere near as many as usual. He seems more alert, cheerful, pleasant and articulate. So much more like the son we lost all those years ago. My family have all noticed the difference as well. At times we have felt like saying "it's so lovely to see you again". Please God, he continues to improve. This weekend inspired me to write "Lost and Found".

Lost and found

Lost and found describes things well
Found nine years on from a voyage to hell
We marvel at the way you've coped
To have you back is more than we'd hoped
For years we had glimpses now and again
These glimpses gave us even more pain
We'd reach out then see you disappear
So many times, year after year
Lost in the horror, sadness and pain
You'd try to break through it time and again
You finally made it, clawed your way through
At last we can see a future for you

Words can never explain how proud we are
To battle so hard, to come so far
To talk together, sheer luxury

More so than ever we thought it would be
You stand before us safe and sound
Lost for years, at long last found
Your voyage over the battle won
Welcome back Christian, we've missed you son.

Where there's a will, there's a way

Where there's a will, there's always a way
My will was to write this story one day
It may help other families who've given up hope
To try to show them how we learned to cope
To spill it all out and help show them the way
To help them go on to another day

I merely existed for almost nine years
Through eternal despair and through so many tears
I felt I'd been wounded with nowhere to go
So hard to accept recovery so slow
I watched over my son with his sadness so rife
Constantly prayed he'd get back his life

I'd have given up everything to set him free
I'd have coped far better had it happened to me
I'd never have dreamt after nine long years
That we'd begin to see an end to our fears
So families out there who are struggling to cope
The one thing you'll need in abundance is hope

All you patients out there

I wrote this poem because I'm angry. I find it hard to take in that there are people out there who could possibly be helped by Clozaril. I know our son has got a long way to go, but we can see some improvement. Yes, he still has problems, but they are nowhere near as bad and that is after three weeks. We are also still very cautious. We have learned over the years that this is the best way. If this book helps just one person to fight back then it has all been worth it.

I am not suggesting that this drug will work for everybody, as you will see from this book, Christian has failed to improve on several. I am saying that when things get so bad (see "Mum, Do You Think I Will Ever Be Free?") there is not much left to lose. After all, sanity has already been lost.

All you patients out there

All you patients out there
Who suffer every day
Read this book and learn
It might show you the way
Have the strength to fight back

Fight even though you're ill
Maybe it will help you too

Ask for Clozaril
When our son finally tried it
We'd almost lost our way
In our wildest dreams we never dreamt
He'd ever see this day

After nine long years of suffering
We could never count the cost
Of things our son missed out on
The months, the years he's lost
We must put all that behind us
As he begins a better life
It's pointless looking back now
On all that pain and strife

So read this and believe us
For years our son was ill
Then at last they tried it
Thank God for Clozaril

The seeds of recovery

This one came to me at 3am on 15th November 1999. I lost a lot of sleep over this poem as I kept altering the words. Hopefully I got it right in the end. Seeing Christian improve is a very slow process, but very clear to see. As the poem tries to explain, it is like watching tiny shoots coming through after so many long years. Very subtle and yet very real. We just keep praying that they will turn into strong young plants.

The seeds of sweet recovery

The seeds of sweet recovery
Take root after endless eternity
Growing stronger after so many years
Watered daily by too many tears
Growth that finally provides the key
Unlocking the seeds of recovery.
Tend the rich soil with tired hands
Reap the new harvest and keep making plans
Seeds we planted so long ago
Fed faithfully with love to watch them grow
With hope replenished you make your way
At last looking forward to the next day
No more endless sleep or angry voices
Far less confused and making choices
Gone evil dreams and hallucinations
Far more relaxed without these frustrations

The new drug working slow but sure
Enriching the soil procuring the cure
Rich and nourishing cool dark earth
Encouraging growth and promoting re-birth

So good to see you less paranoid
In a far kinder world and filling the void
Rebuilding your life, a mammoth task
"Where do I begin?" you quietly ask
"At the beginning", I gently suggest
"Don't take on too much, take time to rest
Tread oh so lightly one step at a time
Remember you walk a very fine line".
Tend the rich soil and at last we see
Seeds of sweet recovery

Frustration

Frustration is about just that. I wrote it during Christian's final weeks at Weymarks. He was taken to clubs during the day by various support workers. He really hated going, but his key worker would encourage him to go. He had been on Clozaril for some months and the senior consultant would check with his key worker whether he was attending because he had to be seen to be socialising if he was going to move on to semi-supported care in Kitt Katts. But the hard fact was that he absolutely detested going. I can remember him saying, "Mum, the people are so ill that most of them can't hold a conversation, so how am I expected to socialise with them?" Of course, there are no answers and we found it harder and harder to stay positive because it was really difficult listening to Chris's complaining especially as we also knew exactly where he was coming from.

I don't think it will be all plain sailing, just because Chris is improving. In fact, I think the next few years will be hard. He was so young when he became ill and, of course, Chris hasn't developed at the same rate as he would have done had he not become ill. I can't get my head around the fact that he is almost 27 years of age and, as he can be quite impatient, I absolutely know that he will want to try to make up for virtually losing ten years of his life. Although this seems quite daunting, compared with the past, it will be a piece of cake.

Frustration

Frustration stares you in the face
Just as you thought you'd won the race
You're much improved, but life's unkind
New prospects are so hard to find
Social clubs they take you to
With people far worse off than you
You mix with others with far less hope

It makes you sad, so hard to cope.
The nurses try hard to explain
They know it drives you clean insane
They're aware you should be moving on
They know your battle's almost won
They know it's hard, you're almost there
And shortly you'll be out of care
Grit your teeth and carry on
It's really not for very long
Stare frustrations back in face
And prove that you will win this race
You'll find a job and show us all
And this time we won't see you fall

Needing a friend

I find that isolation is one of the worst aspects of mental illness. When Chris rings and says, 'I'm going to the pictures or swimming (alone, of course), it always makes me feel so sad. My sister is the same. I tend not to tell her; lately, she has enough on her plate.

One day he went to a snooker club. He stayed in there alone for about six hours. When he went to pay, he didn't have enough money, as they charged him for a year's membership and, as he stayed in there so long, he owed a lot. He took the money back the next day and he hasn't been back since. Only the other day, he went swimming and an older man had offered to lend Chris his goggles. He said, 'No, that's OK, thanks'. After a while, the man got out and sat overlooking the pool. He beckoned Chris over and asked him, would he like to join him for a drink, which Chris declined. What worried me was that Chris was convinced that the man was just lonely. In fact, he said, 'I think he was like me, Mum. He just wanted someone to talk to.'

Chris also said that he's often felt like talking to people and these are the things that, even though we're well aware that he is much better than he was, we still find very sad.

Needing a friend

Loneliness engulfs you, you need a friend by your side
You keep it well under wraps, you've always had too much pride
You go to the pictures alone, the thought always makes me sad
I often think of the past and remember the friends you once had

They gradually fell by the wayside, they've forgotten that you exist
They don't know how much you've needed them or how much they've been missed
All getting on with their lives, enjoying the fun and the pleasure
As the years roll by, unlike you, they'll have plenty of memories to treasure

Yet I know you'll keep soldiering on, with a will that's unwilling to bend
How do I shake off the sadness of knowing you need a friend?

Opportunities

This poem refers to the conversations Chris and I have regarding his future. I must try to be more positive, as he so wants to go forward with his life now. It is so difficult when you have seen someone suffer so much for so long. But, on the other hand, I must learn to encourage him in whatever he decides to do.

Opportunities

"Opportunities that's what I need
Opportunities, are we agreed?"
"Yes, of course but don't take on too much"
"But I'm sick of relying on you as a crutch"
But don't go from the ridiculous to the sublime
Please try to take one day at a time
You've been through so much try to give yourself space
"Mum I've waited for years I must up the pace

I'm twenty-five now not seventeen
There's a great big void in the years in between
A great empty space that I must fill"
But you cannot afford to make yourself ill
"How come you cope? Why aren't I the same?
I'm just like a cripple but emotionally lame"
Try to be patient for just a bit longer
Allow yourself time to heal and get stronger
"Opportunities that's what I need
Opportunities are we agreed?"

At last I agree to give up the fight
I step aside and pray that you're right
And that opportunities are what you need
With fingers crossed at least we're agreed

Fellow sufferers

I'd like at this point to tell you about some other families I have met along the way. I have asked their permission and, of course, like me, they would like to help because of their own suffering. I will not mention any names though.

One lady took her son to hospital in sheer desperation. He began drinking to drown the voices. He would sometimes smoke two cigarettes at a time and stub them out on his mattress. She couldn't sleep because he was ranting and raving all night. One Sunday morning she took him to hospital to be told "take him home, we haven't a bed for him"

Another young man became so ill that he stabbed someone because he firmly believed that this person was living within his own skin. His parents were told that he was one of the worst cases they had seen. The only drug in

11 years that has controlled his horrendous symptoms is Clozaril. He has in fact been stable on it for a number of years, but, tragically, he and his family will pay a high price for the rest of their lives for the fact that this young man's terrible illness led to such dreadful circumstances. I think of this lad and I hear his mother saying "he was the worst case of psychosis they'd seen and now look at him, stable at long last."

Yet another mother that I speak to on a regular basis is terrified that her 28 year old son will eventually kill himself. He believes that he is Elvis Presley's son and that there are people trying to kill him, in his words, "as they killed my father". This lady doesn't know where to turn and in the back of my mind I'm constantly wondering would Clozaril help him. Eventually, he was tried on Clozaril and for the first four weeks, he showed all the same signs of improvement as Christian. His mum and I had lots of conversations about how lucky we were to have managed to get them both on it. One evening she rang me in tears, saying he'd been taken into hospital and the Clozaril monitoring service had put him on red alert, as his white blood count had dropped dramatically. This means that the drug has to be withdrawn immediately, as it can be very dangerous to the immune system. The whole family were devastated.

They were told that he could never go on it again. We couldn't imagine how they must have felt to see him get so well and then have that happen. It goes back to the old saying 'There's always someone worse off'.

I am well aware of the fact that there is no cure for schizophrenia. I also have finally accepted that my son will never be as well as he would have been, or achieve what he might have done, but I hope readers can see that he doesn't go through that hell any more and we often say that, over the years, we have wondered if the life he had was really worth living. Christian's quality of life we feel, bearing in mind that we lived with this daily for seven and a half years when he was living at home, has changed dramatically for the better, and we no longer feel terrified of what we all might have to go through next.

In conclusion, these are the questions I constantly ask myself: Why in the name of God does it keep going on? Why are people still dying, either through suicide or the desperate actions of a very sick person? Why don't general practitioners, practice nurses and other members of the primary health care teams know enough (not just about schizophrenia), but also about the need to show these poor souls and their families the compassion and the respect that they so very obviously need and, of course, deserve? Will it ever change? Please God—one day.

Will I ever be able to mention that word schizophrenia without seeing that look I all too often get, a mixture of horror and lack of understanding rolled into one? If and when I ever get an answer to these questions, I will be able to rest, so remember:

Try to learn
Don't turn away
Who knows it might
Be you one day

One thing I know, the memories of these families and the ever nagging, wondering how things are with them will never leave me. It's not possible, there are many more that I could mention, I've just picked out a few.

Life without poetry

This poem is about the panic I feel when I think that it's all going to come to an end one day. I wonder how I will cope, as I remember how I felt before it all started. The bottom line is, no matter how much we have been affected by something there is only so much that can be written. It seems as if it could be drying up as the poem suggests. Perhaps I will take some time off and then start again with a different subject. We will just have to wait and see. To be honest I don't think this will ever happen because, as you can see, this is not about me having a talent for writing, it is about far more than that.

Life without poetry

Has it finally stopped flowing, must I start to let go?
Has it almost diminished and how will I know?
But you're not in control, in fact it controls you
Don't shake your head, you know that it's true
Is it parched and dried up like a disused well
Will it flow once more freely, perhaps time will tell
It's served its purpose and helped with my rage
Soothing my soul as it reaches each page
Trusting and loyal like a long lost friend
Hard to contemplate life, if it's come to and end
Flowing out passively night after night
Healing my wounds after each endless fight
I try to visualise life without it one day
Will there be a price that I have to pay?
Will I start to feel lonely as I did before?
I can't force it to stay, will there be any more
But you're not in control you know it controls you
I nod in agreement knowing it's true

They say all good things must come to an end
But I fear I'll be lost without my best friend
Without it whatever will my life be
Must prepare for a life without poetry

Fighting back

I've been trying for weeks to think of a way to conclude this book. I've used the title "Fighting Back". Fighting back explains how I have viewed the illness as a monster, and how before I began writing, I was defeated by it time and time again, but not anymore. Now at last I'm, fighting back.

Fighting back

I came face to face with a monster
I was weak and it invaded my life
It caused so much devastation
As it hacked at me with a knife
It attacked my son and dragged him away
It left me not knowing would I see the day
My son would return from his journey to hell
There was no way of knowing, no way I could tell
I felt its breath so very close
Hot and putrid as it came through it's nose
So often it reared its ugly head
Filling my soul with fear and dread
I just submitted I see that now
It sensed my weakness just knew somehow
Time and again I just let it abuse
Desperate for revenge with no weapons to use
Just a shell of a person filled with fright
Far too weak to put up a fight

Then God gave me the weapons to help me fight back
At last I'm prepared for every attack
Armed with a sword and a very large shield
I'll start fighting back and no longer yield
With courage renewed I'll raise to its height
I'm ready, I'm willing, I'm able to fight
At last my weakness has turned into fury
I've been given the strength to write this story
When it gets too close I'll give it a whack
After all of these years I'm "Fighting Back"

One part of all this I've never been sure of is the tiredness. Sometimes I think it is the illness that causes it and other times I think it is one of the effects of these very powerful medications.

Chris gets confused sometimes and he will stare at me in amazement when I'm doing the housework, or he'll say "mum, how does dad keep on working without getting tired? I only work a few hours and I feel so very tired."

He does get better as the day goes on (as we all do), but the first thing I notice when he gets up, irrespective of the time, is the tiredness. It does seem all consuming. I suppose it's like everything else, he's become used to it after ten years.

Social Services rang today

I've met quite a few social workers during these years and I've come to the conclusion that those who I feel do their jobs best are the older ones who are married with a family. It's not a matter of criticising the younger ones, it's just that, on this type of job, I feel that the more experience they've had of life, the better equipped they are in this type of work. Qualifications are all well and good, but there's nothing as educational as life itself.

An incident that springs to mind was about a year ago. Chris was waiting for his final assessment meeting before being transferred from Weymarks, which was 24-hour care, to his present home, Kitt Katts, which is 12-hour care. His social worker, a young man not much older than himself, had some conflicting opinions with Christian's CPN. He let me know that he didn't like the CPN very much, also a young man about the same age as Christian. Apparently, the social worker makes the decision whether or not the CPN attends this final meeting and, because of the conflict between them, he decided not to invite the CPN along to accompany my son. I was very angry because it was blatantly obvious that the social worker was ignoring the need of the patient (Chris) and putting his own prejudices first. My son should have been his first priority, not his pathetic protest against the CPN.

By time the meeting took place, this particular social worker had left, but still the CPN was not invited. The evening of the day of the meeting, Chris rang and said that he felt as if he'd had a straightjacket on all day. He was very upset. He had gone into the room and the first question he was asked was, 'Are you violent?' Weymarks is just a house in an ordinary road. There are children living two doors away. I was furious to say the least. Why hadn't they done their homework? I've told Chris that if he's ever asked this question again, he should reply, 'No, I'm not, are you?'

First thing next morning, I rang social services and said I'd been wondering if they knew anything about mental illness. They sent a social worker to Weymarks to apologise to Christian, but the damage was done. I must add, the most of the NHS care that Christian has received has been good and the same is true of social services. Christian's current social worker is excellent and I know that she tries her best for all of us.

The point of all this is that the very first priority should always be the patient and those who work with them should consider the affect of their actions on people as vulnerable as my son.

Social Services rang today

Social Services rang today with your social worker's name
Social services rang today to us they all seem the same

Young articulate and straight out of college
Of mental illness will he have any knowledge?

Or is it all learned from books drummed right into his brain
How can he possibly know what it's like to go insane

He's reserved us a place on Tuesday, we'll go to the centre to meet
He'll speak in very hushed tones and nervously shuffle his feet

Will he understand our son, will he treat him like a statistic?
We must try not to get irate though we feel we could go ballistic

We'll discuss your precarious future, at present you're living in care
Could you manage to live alone, or is it better that you share?

He'll ask us if you're stable and reliable with your medication
Do you still tend to stay in bed, any improvement with motivation?

Social services rang today with your social workers name
Social services rang today and we're tired of playing their game

Policy No: FB228727

I joined a health scheme at work it seemed a good idea. If you had to go into hospital you would subsequently be paid so much per night. I signed for it without reading all the terms and conditions. They eventually sent me a copy of their terms and conditions and when I read them I was horrified to see that the same rules do not apply to people suffering from mental illnesses. I find this totally unacceptable. I really can't see what difference it possibly makes. No one wants to be ill, whether it mentally or physically, but they make a definite line between the two conditions. Needless to say, I cancelled the policy and told them why.

Policy No: FB228727

I cancel my policy forthwith
Since reading your terms and conditions
How can you segregate people
In such a vulnerable position

Should they suffer from sugar diabetes
The benefits are very good
But not so with mental illness
But I feel that it should

It made me so very angry
What difference does it make
It's not their fault that it happens
But they're treated like a fake

A neuro-biological disorder
Transmitters gone wrong in the brain
So it stems from a physical cause
And causes emotional pain

But these people are penalised
They're at the bottom of life's pile
But these things don't ever get questioned
Not even once in a while

My son suffers from mental illness
He has done for many years
You've no idea of the struggle
The heartache or the tears

I don't think you'll understand me
But I'm praying for the day

For these people things will improve
So I'll just keep chipping away

So I expect you to cancel this policy
As I find it too hard to conceive
And I'd sooner go without it

Will you ever give up the fight

I joined my local library to see if they had any books about schizophrenia. They had two; one called 'Tell me I'm here' and the other, 'Monkey's Uncle', which they told me wasn't even a true story. They were unable to supply the latter and, after a very long wait, in which they had to search for it in other areas, I managed to get 'Tell me I'm here' by Anne Deveson. This book tells the tragic story of her son, who finally committed suicide at the age of 24 years, after six years of suffering. I wrote this poem after reading the book, because this was our worst nightmare, Chris giving up the fight as Jonathan Deveson did.

Will you ever give up the fight?

I ask myself every day
How much more can you take?
I've often felt tempted to say
You say you often feel old
Which doesn't surprise me at all
I've watched you pick yourself up
After every relentless fall

Will you ever give up the fight?
I can't bear to think that you will
I've just read about someone who did
He got tired of being ill
At 24 years old, two years younger than you
After years of mental pain
Unable to carry life through

But who are we to decry him
He wasn't just making a fuss
Would we be able to cope?
If it happened to one of us
I pray you'll carry on
I suppose it's selfish of me
I can't think of life without you
What kind of life would that be?

There must be a point to it all
Perhaps one we'll discover one day
A reason for all your suffering
Such a price you had to pay

Will you ever give up the fight?
We'll just have to wait and see
We pray every night that you won't
Your dad, your brother and me

Conflicting opinions

I asked my mum the other day if she believed, as I do, that my sister's prayer was heard. But she thinks I was driven to write all this by the pain that I'd kept inside for years and years. She also said that she feels had I not been able to get all this out of my system, I too would have suffered a breakdown. She said it was just like a pressure cooker letting out all the steam. It had released the pain and with it the anxiety.

Readers will of course draw their own conclusions and I'm sure there will be many conflicting opinions. I will always believe that the prayer was heard and acted upon. This is not because I am a religious person, it's purely what I feel inside.

Buy one get one free

Last night I was watching a play on ITV called "Little Bird". It was about a couple who were trying to adopt a child. They were given a form by social services in which they were asked would they consider adopting a child with certain disabilities, one of them being schizophrenia. The husband said "That would be good, two for the price of one". I find it hard to believe that statements like this are still being made at prime viewing time where so many people are yet again being given the wrong information. Then yet again another night I woke at 2.30am and started to write.

The lady who played the part of the social worker dealing with the case was Amanda Burton and as I was putting my pen and paperwork away, I was thinking about all the other parts I had seen her play. I remember she played the part of a pathologist in a BBC series called "Silent Witness". This was the inspiration for the poem. It made me wonder how much research was done into the subject of schizophrenia prior to the filming of this programme. Judging by what was said, none at all. Yet I thought they always did extensive research into any medical condition so as not to give people false information. Yet again, it seems that, for mental disorders, this is not important. It's only schizophrenia after all.

Buy one get one free

I can't believe I didn't know
But I didn't have a clue
Now answer me with honesty
Is it just the same for you?
Whilst I enjoyed my life
Engulfed in ignorant bliss

I swear I didn't know
I was blind to all of this

I've had a mental illness
Why on earth did I not see?
So many people suffering
And so much more than me
I still can't quite believe it
The writing helps me cope
And if it spreads the word
It at least provides some hope

The more we learn of this condition
The more we share our fear
The quicker we'll dispel the myths
At last make people hear
If reporters read this book
Will they change the way they write?
Could they show overdue compassion
So we'll see an end in sight

Then when we read the tabloids
Words like psycho won't be used
And with this fresh approach
They'll no longer be abused
An end to all the stigma
Will help them bear the pain
And the words that you are reading
Will not have been in vain

Their voice

Out of all of the poems I have written I think this one is my favourite. It explains how pleased I am to find something positive in the midst of negativity. Writing has been my only defence against schizophrenia. Without it I would have been consumed by it.

I've also been pleased to pay a very small tribute to a handful of sufferers I've met along the way. Some of them don't even have families to support them, the help and support they give one another has amazed Paul and I.

I will never forget the kindness they have shown Christian. It gave us a lot of comfort in the two and a half years he spent in rehab because we knew they, along with the staff would look after him.

Their voice

I've been a silent witness
For far too many years
I've met many other sufferers
Cried many futile tears
Not just for my own son
But for the others he has known
As I've watched them battle bravely
My respect for them has grown

Now ten years from the start
This is what I find
The one's that lose themselves
Are the one's who lose their mind
I've sat in rehab centres
I've watched them shuffle past
I've prayed to God that one day
They'll find some peace at last

There must be someway I could help them
It seemed ludicrous to me
I've marvelled at their strength
Their sheer tenacity
Embedded in my memory are Sid and Des and Paul
Many more than I can mention
I respect them one and all

Along with dedicated nurses who've listened endlessly
To irrational fears and worries
So very patiently
For years I felt so helpless
Was there nothing I could do?
Then a miracle occurred
And the writing filtered through

I thank God I started writing
He's given me a choice
No more a silent witness
I'll try to be their voice

Humility

When I started writing this book, I was desperate for people to see what my son was going through. But as it's gone on, I feel it is apparent that I have also been very touched by all the others I've met along the way. It's not just about my family, it's about all the millions of people all over the world whose lives have been effected by schizophrenia. Paul and I often think about the families that must have been torn apart by it's effects because if one parent understood and the other didn't it would of course be disastrous. I think it would be fair to say that because of the deep feelings it has so obviously conjured up within me, I've made it my personal mission, I dare say some would say obsession, to try to dispel the myths. At least, it's something positive, and if it doesn't help to justify why this has happened to my son, it helps me because if it helps other people it will at least serve a purpose.

Humility

Will it help to dispel the myths
I can only pray it might
Will people be willing to learn
Can we see an end in sight
Will reading this help them to see
This can happen to anyone
So never lose sight of this
It could be your daughter or son

Never dreamt it would happen to us
Thought it only happened to others
So do try to take this in
All you fathers or mothers
We must help them stand up for their rights
And insist on the best medications
Please don't suffer in silence for years
Scared to ask for some explanations

One day people with mental illness
Will be shown the respect they are due
And no longer be treated as outcasts
Not even by a few
Will it help to dispel the myths
Till at long last all of us see
That people with mental illness
Can teach us humility

No props

This poem is about the fact that if you are blind, in a wheelchair or even deaf you have a small advantage over people with mental illness. Please don't take this the wrong way, I'm not saying that it is any easier to deal with than say, blindness. I would never dream of forming an opinion on something I know nothing about, but the small advantage is that, because of wheelchairs, white sticks, and hearing aids, there is something that visually shows these people have disabilities. It is not so with any form of mental illness. Of course, this in turn causes problems. Sometimes I've met people from work at the weekend at Lakeside and on Monday morning they've said ,"that wasn't your son who's ill with you on Saturday was it?" Looking at Christian you would never know. When I watch him go into the warehouse to work I think "God, they don't know just how hard it is for him to do just four hours work. These feelings are what made me want to write this one.

I read an article about a man in America. His name is Frederick Friese. He is now a psychotherapist. At the hospital, he was admitted to when he first became ill years before, at one time he wore a sign around his neck which read "Please be careful how you speak to me as I am very sensitive and words can hurt me. I suffer from an illness called schizophrenia". I found this sad and amazing.

No props

There's nothing to outwardly show
So I couldn't expect you to know
He doesn't stand out in a crowd
His voice tends to be quiet not loud
As I watch him go in with the rest
Only we know how hard is the test
As there isn't a label to tell
The times that my son's been to hell
If he wore one at least you could see
Just how hard his life can be
But he seems just the same as you
So it's hard to believe it's true
But believe me beneath the illusion
He can battle with total confusion
So look deeply beneath the veneer
And with patience it will become clear
Don't be too proud to be taught
He desperately needs your support
Be generous and try not to ration
Understanding, support and compassion
With all this to help him along
Given time he will become strong
If you can manage to pull our the stops
There won't be a need for the props.

People with schizophrenia

This poem explains my need to justify what I was like for years and I must say that I feel much better for it. I was no different from the people who stare at me blankly when I talk about Christian. I can remember taking him for his injection at Sunnyside when he was about 18 years old, and I was talking to a lady who was with her daughter. I can remember saying, "is this your daughter?" as if the poor girl didn't exist. I often cringe when I think of how they both must have felt. I know that with the knowledge I have now, I would be angry if somebody did it to me. Once someone asked if my son was a schizophrenic and I replied, "No my son is a young man who suffers from a condition called schizophrenia". I hope they got the message and will re-phrase what they have to say in the future.

My only defence in all this is that I feel things should have been explained in far more detail to us much earlier on and, although I read all the leaflets supplied by NSF, SANE and MIND and also various books like "Living With Schizophrenia", I couldn't find anything anywhere written from a family point of view. My sister is a prolific reader and she also tried to find one and that's another reason to try to get this published. I do hope that people in the same situation will find my work helpful in some way.

People with schizophrenia

My son suffers from schizophrenia
I'm frequently heard to say
I try to educate people
I feel I must show them the way
People do tend to get embarrassed
They're not sure how to react
I sympathise with their reasons
When I say it so matter of fact
It's hard to believe it's me
After covering it up for years
Never daring to share my secret
Harbouring so many fears
I was so petrified
So for years I hid it away
"My son suffers from his nerves"
I was often heard to say

To this day I still feel guilty
I was weak for such a long time
How wrong to hide it away
As if he'd committed a crime
I tell them I'm proud of my son
I often use his name
I'm rid of the feelings of secrecy
Along with the feelings of shame
They stem from not enough learning
But it's only fair to say
If schizophrenia hadn't touched my life
I'd surely be the same way

My reasons for writing our story
The conclusion to ten long years
Is to try to dispel the stigma
See an end to the frustrated fears
So try not to be like I was
Ashamed, bewildered and sad

Then hopefully with education
Things won't be quite so bad

Lets talk openly about schizophrenia
Let's share our worries and fears
No more deep dark secrets
No more lonely tears
By bringing it out in the open
We will gain respect from the media
And the public will know a bit more
About people with schizophrenia

Schizophrenia's year

Since I've realised that this isn't just about us, I've felt the need to write more and more about the plight of others far less fortunate than Christian. I have it on good authority that there are many young people out there who haven't had a medication preview for years. I know that Clozaril isn't a wonder drug, but I can only quote what I've seen myself and that is that my son has improved on it a great deal and I would love to see others given the same chance and then at least we would know.

I've been told that a lot of people living out in the community are not reliable with medication or having the blood tested on a regular basis, and of course it would be wonderful if Clozaril were available in the form of a depot injection so that they didn't have this responsibility. But I've seen Chris improve so much on it that he would be far more likely to take on that responsibility now than he ever would have been on Piportil, because he's nowhere near as confused and the florid symptoms are much better than they were. So it's a case of the chicken and the egg. Until Chris went on Clozaril, he didn't get on buses and the couple of times he did, he came home distressed because he thought the people at the bus stops and on the buses were talking about him. I'm not taking anything away from the dedicated people who have helped him, but even they would agree with me about the difference the medication change has made. In fact, one of the nurses said he's a walking advert for Clozaril. I'm sure some people will read this and say that, in their opinion, Chris's recovery is due to the fact that writing has been therapeutic to me. That is partly true, but the right drug is so very important and our story proves this.

Could this be schizophrenias year?

Is there anyone out there to hear
Could this be schizophrenia's year?
There are too many patients due
A full medication review
But no one seems to hear them
Ever the silent voice
Sentenced to half a life

Should they not be given the choice?
To try drugs that work, like Clozaril
Could they not be given a trial?
Don't leave them out there to rot
At the bottom of life's pile

Things are better for people with AIDS
And I'm not suggesting that's wrong
But people with schizophrenia
Have been patient for far too long
If it improves their lives by a little
Would it not be money well spent
If it allowed them a little more peace
Would their lives not be more content

Our son has been very lucky
We've been here to help with this fight
But there's many far less fortunate
Alone in their dreadful plight
Will these words ever manage to help them
Is there any one out there to hear
We're still within the Millennium
Will it be schizophrenia's year?

And so it goes on

Ironically, as I was just completing this book, the newspapers were full of the story of Michael Abrams who broke into George Harrison's home and stabbed him ten times. Of course, it made a bigger story than usual because it involved a famous celebrity. I paid particular attention to detail and yet another all too familiar story began to unfold. It's a known fact that lots of young people, including Christian, use illegal drugs during the onset of schizophrenia, looking for a way to alleviate symptoms. From what I could gather without knowing all the facts, it does look as if this was the case here.

Even though Michael's mother tried to get him help and even though several psychiatrists saw him, it was systematically assumed that he was suffering from drug-induced psychosis and so, inevitably, the pot eventually boils over and consequently causes mayhem. It was more by luck than judgement that no one died.

Tragically, now Michael Abrams and his entire family, face a very bleak future and the final diagnosis some nine years too late is, of course, schizophrenia. As I watched his mother on TV saying "My son is a lovely lad, but at the time that this occurred he was very sick" the tears ran down my face and I wondered how may people were saying, "How on earth can she say that about some one who has committed such a dreadful crime (son or no son)"?

I would like to say at this point how much I admired George Harrison's son for having the intelligence and decency to say on TV that his family have every sympathy for anyone who is suffering from this tragic illness.

In conclusion, please ask yourselves if you really believe that this would have still happened if this young man had received the professional care he so desperately needed. I for one do not think so.

Found myself

Found myself is a poem I really enjoyed writing because it does have a positive ending. Even though Chris still has a few bad times you can see that he is recovering. Sometimes he does take a few steps back, but he very quickly gets over it and he doesn't dwell on things. It's quite amazing how positive he is, if ever we get a little despondent. I read some of the poems from years ago and then we say "God, this is nothing. Just look at what we used to have to cope with" and this is very helpful.

Found myself

Injured bird—broken wing
Used to fly—used to sing
Gains some height, soars up high
Drops like a stone from a clear blue sky
A decade of meaningless isolation
Searching for a long lost motivation
Facing relentless journey blind
With lost emotions muddled mind
Dampened passion sadly lost
Soldier on at any cost

Shattered future—endless trying
Futility and hopeless crying
Racing mind that's starved of sleep
Tenacious hope—crops to reap
Gritted teeth determines choices
Amidst a sea of angry voices
Pointless, senseless years of fear
Won't let you rob another year

Wing starts healing, confidence found
Takes me up to safer ground
A decade of suffering in the past
Found myself at long, long last.

We're the voice

Can you hear us? We're the voice
It's time you gave us all a choice
Anti-psychotics, depots, potions
A wilderness of lost emotions
One whole decade can't believe
Misspent youth we can't retrieve
Do they say things to annoy ya'

This one's great for paranoia
Under white coats lurk the thugs
No you take them stick your drugs
You know there's no more we can do
Then go to hell it's up to you
Legs like jelly mouth so dry
Tears that sting behind the eye
Medicine ball replaces head
Feels so heavy filled with lead
Live in hope die in despair
Can you hear us? You out there

We need good drugs to make us well
Sick of years we've spent in hell
Days and months and years we've lost
Then they tell us it's the cost
Need to laugh love and play
There's one last thing we need to say
Ask yourself if it were you
Would you be ranting and raving too
It's time you gave us all a choice
Can you hear us? We're the voice?

Moving mountains

The time has come at long last
There's no more left to say
My greatest wish of all
Is it might help to show you the way
To treat people with schizophrenia
That you'll start to understand
That this life isn't what they wanted
And certainly not what they'd planned
They'll be spared a little thought
For the courage they're forced to use
In the wake of all their suffering
They'll no longer feel abused
These words have served a purpose
It won't have all been in vain
And with the wisdom of fresh understanding
They'll find it easier to bear the pain
With the promise of new medications
And the hope that they might improve
Maybe as the Millennium closes
We will see the mountains move

Could I be doing more?

I would hate readers to think that there is a drug available to control the symptoms of this illness to such an extent that their loved one is completely as he or she would have been had this illness not occurred, although, if it is controlled by a suitable drug in the early stages, this is possible. I do feel that, as carers for years, we've learned enough to say that Clozaril has proved to be the best drug that our son has been on and that his suffering was cut down considerably right from the start, and I think readers have learned enough by reading about it to know that our lives have improved.

Lastly, I'd like to say to parents in this situation, please don't be too hard on yourselves. Paul and I have come to see that, with all the will and love in the world, sadly, there is only so much we can do. I do hope that parents will have learned enough from our story to stand up for their rights and insist on a medication change, if you feel your son or daughter is not improving. Then, at least like us, you will enjoy the comfort of knowing that you've done all you can and will be free at last from the ever nagging question, could I be doing more?

The fog is clearing

This poem is about the many times that Christian tries to find a reason for all the years of pain. I try, constantly, to tell him to look to the future and put it all behind him. I talk to him about all the millions of people who are suffering from all sorts of things, not just this illness, but still he tries to rationalise it by trying to find out what's caused it all to happen. I can only hope that, with time, he will just accept it, and who knows how long it will take. It's not exactly an easy thing to accept. Again, it's a process we must all go through with him. At least, it's another indication that the fog is clearing for him.

The fog is clearing

Mum I keep feeling angry
Will we ever measure the cost?
When I think of the hurt it's caused us
The decade that's all been lost
Do you think my accident caused it?
We've gone over this all before
We'll really never know Chris
What's brought it all to the fore

You must have been predisposed
Perhaps it was in your genes
I mean I've had a mental illness
"But I don't see what all that means"
"Maybe it was the mugging
I'll never forget that day

He gets a year behind bars
And leaves me the price to pay
Something must have caused it
What do you think it could be?
When I hurt my finger at Palmers?"
Chris it's no good asking me
You just have to learn to accept it
Like all painful things in this life
We all know it can't be easy
It's the sharpest edge of the knife
It's time to stop looking back
The worst part is now in the past
Try harder to keep looking forwards
The future is brighter at last

"But mum, I'll always wonder
It's taken so much of me"
But thank God things are improving
That's blatantly clear to see
Try not to be bitter and angry
That's purely a waste of time
The fog is beginning to clear now
Eventually things will be fine.

Every now and then

Now and then is about life now and how, occasionally, I see Chris go back there. I can't explain things any better than that. I wish I couldn't see it and I'm probably the only person who can. Only another mother will know what I mean. I have to be extremely careful not to be engulfed by his suffering, as I've learned enough to know that it is totally pointless.

Every now and then

Every now and then I see you count the cost,
Reflecting on the past, taking stock of what you've lost
Your face looks fraught with fear, your eyes fill up with tears
Ghosts come back to haunt you as you grieve for wasted years

Season after season, stark futility
Important lessons we have learned, first in line; humility
Every now and then, I see you looking sad
A giant void replaces all the fun you should have had

The fragrance of fine perfume, nights of endless passion
A decade of sheer pleasure; my heart aches with compassion
I feel the cauldron pulling me, but I can't go there again
I must protect my feelings, I must not feel your pain

I'll keep looking to the future, the past is hard to comprehend
Things are looking better, except for now and then

Coming home

This is one that I thought I'd never get to write. Seeing our son so ill for so many years, I often wondered if he would have to stay in care indefinitely. I hope you agree that this is a very good note to end on and it proves that miracles really can happen if you wait long enough, and pray hard enough and, of course, love each other enough.

Chris rang my Mum to say that he had some good news. When I got to Mum's at 2pm Thursday 7th December 2000, she said I must ring him back at Kitt Katts. After the phone call my mum said, "surely that will prompt you to write another poem" to which I replied "no mother, the book is well and truly finished, I've actually written **The End**". So I've got my mum to blame for this one because I woke up at 1.30am and there it was "Coming Home" I rang her Friday morning and read it to her.

Coming home

Mum, I'm coming home
What a great surprise
I'm almost lost for words and tears spring to my eyes
They'll help me after Christmas
To make it on my own
My heart swells up with pride
For the courage you have shown
They all say I've done well
That I've coped remarkably
Thank God for drugs like Clozaril
It's helped to set me free
I could either get a flat
Or come back to live with you
The joy within these words
I can't believe it's true
We never thought we'd hear them
Not even in our dreams
Only we know how you've battled
Only we know what this means

It's a dream come true for all of us
The nightmare finally ends
Mum I'll miss the people
I've made some real good friends
But it's time now I moved on
Right away from care
I won't forget these years though
At times so hard to bear

Mum I'm coming home
How magical that sounds
Our son is coming home
The one we lost and found

Dedicated people

I can't finish this book without writing about all the dedicated people who have helped our son and many others and of course the families that are also so involved in all of this.

People like Jim, Christian's occupational therapist who, for his two and a half year stay in rehab, took him swimming (for which he got a certificate), woodwork classes, and nature walks. Jim knew exactly what buttons to push to help boost his continually flagging confidence. Nurses, doctors and care workers and, even now at Kitt Katts, Pam and her team who have taken over where Weymarks left off, using exactly the same tactics, respect, compassion, and patience, which in time, lots of time, obviously moves mountains.

As you know after reading this book, a very very big part in Christian's recovery is undoubtedly due to Clozaril. After being a carer for all those years, you would have been blind not to see the changes taking place. This, together with the support he's had from so many good people and a family who love him dearly, has proved to us that miracles do happen.

Why not me?

Why has this happened to us?
I've asked myself too many times
I've yet to come up with an answer
Yet I've searched for years for some signs
Why has this happened to us?
We are people who do no wrong
Should we never question our plight
Should we just keep soldiering on

But the answer remains the same
In fact, nobody ever knows why
They say it's pointless to ask 'Why me'
Just the same, as it's pointless to cry
I must change my way of thinking
I'm sure you will agree
The best way to answer this question
Is to answer it, "Why not me?"

Every mother's nightmare

This morning I was paid a visit by Julia Billecij, who is a manager of the patient monitoring group of Clozaril. Julia works for Novartis, the manufacturers of Clozaril. I was very pleased, as Julia wants me to go to Manchester with her in March to read some of my work to 100 senior consultants in the hope that our story may encourage more consultants to try their patients on Clozaril. Of course, I'm only too happy to help because this drug has helped Chris so much.

Around 6pm Chris rang and I told him all about it, as I tell him anything that involves the book. If you remember I've written an article about the fact that I've often wondered if, as the brain is obviously damaged by this disease some parts of it become more developed to compensate. I'll explain what I mean by telling you about the phone call. As I was telling him rather excitedly that I was going to Manchester by plane (my first time) of all the things he said, "God mum, that's strange because last night I dreamt I was in a book shop and I was looking at a section of books entitled "Every Mother's Nightmare" I said, "But that's the title of the book that tells the tragic story of the abduction of Jamie Bulger. Chris said, "Yes I know that, but since I've started to get better, I've often thought about all the trouble I've been to you and dad and that was the context of my dream. That title was referring to me and not the book about Jamie Bulger". Again I found this so strange just as it seems some good is coming out of all this work, Christian has yet another strange dream, it's as if we are connected in some strange way.

Lessons learned

Although we've suffered years of pain
None of them were wasted
Emotions in a stormy sea
Brought salty tears we tasted
The suffering that we've witnessed
Brought lessons to be learned
To journey on to the mountain top
And to leave no stone unturned

For the people who were there for us
We won't forget your care
Sweet comfort you all gave us
Just in knowing you were there
So we'll treat it as a learning curve
For at last it's plain to see
The lesson to be learned from this
Is to have humility

The one thing I've tried to do when writing this book is to be honest about everything I've written. I'm now going to give readers an update on how things are at the moment in time.

Christmas was quite difficult, probably because Chris was going out more than usual. At my work's Christmas meal he could not manage to eat the dinner and asked to go home within three quarters of an hour of getting there. Of course, he spent a lot of time at home, which has led to him having some problems going back to Kitt Katts.

I always think that it must be very difficult being at home for half the week and working and then going back to a care home where the other residents have problems, and I think he's finding it quite hard to adapt to this. He's had a few symptoms, but it hasn't stopped him from going to work. He's very determined to keep his job.

A Christian approach for a new understanding

The following poems, Schizophrenia, Learn, Share and For a New Understanding, have been written to try to promote a better understanding of mental illness. It's the only thing I can do to try to help. I find it hard that, in 2001, attitudes to mental illness still seem to belong to the dark ages. Much of this is due to the media. They rarely report the number of suicides connected to mental illness, but give plenty of coverage if someone who is acutely ill, launches an attack on innocent bystanders. They use emotive words, such as 'Nutter', 'Schizo' and 'Psycho'.

In the past two weeks, our local paper has been full of letters from people opposing flats being built near them to house people with mental illnesses. Where do they expect them to live? If a person has cancer or MS, everyone is sympathetic and there are lots of visitors. It is not so with mental illness, almost as though most people don't class it as an illness.

I decided to run a survey and some of the things people have said are hard to believe. 'Is he violent', 'How did he catch it', 'I've every sympathy, but I wouldn't want one living next door, thank you' are just a few of the responses. After seeing your own child go to hell and back and trying so desperately to work and live a normal life, to hear such comments causes so much pain and heartache.

Schizophrenia

White hot terror surrounds it, schizophrenia the sound of the word
When this label was chosen, they made sure it was heard
It strikes fear in the very soul, even though it remains well hidden
Buried beneath layers of fear, almost as if it's forbidden
I've always wanted to change it to anything other than this
It conjures up mental pictures of a deep, dark, endless abyss
And yet a decade on, it can frighten me no more
I've found peace through understanding and bringing it to the fore
By trying to educate others in my need to let it all out
In the hope that they will learn what this condition is really about

The day will then finally dawn when people at last start seeing
That beneath the label they wear, are some very brave human beings

Learn

Open your eyes and ears, seek and you will find
Read all you can on the subject, open your hearts and mind
There is nothing to be scared of, it is an illness the same as the rest
These people need understanding for theirs is the hardest test
This condition is part of life, it's been here for hundreds of years
Causing incalculable suffering and creating rivers of tears
We no longer treat them like witches, burning them all at the stake
Yet attitudes have not changed much, how much do they have to take?
It is high time we all moved on, we must move away from the past
Then maybe with some understanding, who knows perhaps at last
We can pass on our knowledge to our children and even if it takes years
We will finally understand, if we open our eyes and our ears

Share

Families out there like mine whose suffering is hard to measure
Have witnessed schizophrenia, which robbed them of years of pleasure
Come out and tell your stories, educate the media
Help to dispel the myths surrounding schizophrenia
Share your stories with the world is the only way we'll learn
It is within our capabilities to help make attitudes turn

Try not to be like I was, crying my futile tears
Hidden within my boundaries for too many wasted years
The way forward is ours for the taking without us how would they see
If we all keep hiding away, understanding can never break free
Break open your painful shackles, help me to spread the word
It is nothing to be ashamed of, let understanding fly high like a bird

Old myths will go out of the window and people will start to care
So stop hiding within the confusion and come out with me and share

For a new understanding

I dream of a new understanding where people will show compassion
They will gradually change their views, and humility is never on ration
I dream of a new found hope where people will help each other
They will show mental illness respect and finally discover
That respect is the least they deserve, though a very big part it plays
We move on from our ignorant views, gradually changing our ways

We talk openly about mental illness and throw its dark cloak away
Dissolving negativity and keeping confusion at bay
I dream of the day that reporters will change the way that they write
Nutters, Psychos and Schizos are finally kept out of sight

Do you think the day will come, of course it is yet to be seen
I dream of a new understanding, but will it remain a dream?

Moving mountains and the end of a ten year journey

There have been many times when I have thought it would never end. But here it is at the end of a ten year journey starting with "In the Beginning" through to Christian's admittance to "Ward 12, Basildon" following a relapse some seven years later. Part II, starting with my sister's prayer, and then the contrast between Dr Adrianne Reveley and Dr Dean, "good and evil", two people doing the same job, but absolutely poles apart. And so it goes on to taking Dr Reveley's advice and Christian, subsequently, being given Clozaril, which led to "We Saw You This Weekend", "Seeds of Recovery", and "All You Patients Out There". Looking back, after writing "All You Patients Out There", I really don't know how I didn't see that there was more to come, but I didn't.

So there I was preparing to write the conclusion to it all having decided that "Fighting Back" would be the final poem in the story, and that my final summing up would say that the conclusion to it all is that we had finally gained the strength to fight back, and I call it fate if you like. I was watching a play on ITV, and just because of something that was said, yet again I became engulfed in writing. I can only assume that the frustration I feel deep inside was stirred by the conversation that I felt, yet again, was very misleading. See "Buy One Get One Free". This in turn, led to words upon words 2, 3, 4am in the morning. Exactly the same as before, too powerful to ignore.

But this time there was a subtle difference. Parts I and II are, of course, about our son, our family, and our lives. But this part was about all the people out there who have not been as lucky as Christian, and don't have a family to fight for them. In the poem, "Poetry My Saviour", I've written, "Such a powerful experience. But none of it planned, like liquid gold you drip from my hand". I didn't plan any of this; it came to me very gradually and between parts I, II and III, I've been given a break in writing. Am I wrong? Has it been planned? If not by me, by someone or something else? At the end of the day, the readers must make up their own minds. All I can do is tell it as it is and I get very confused myself. All I can say is the power behind it is what amazes me more than anything.

With this realization came relief because I could then see that Chris must have improved a lot for me to be now able to focus my attention on all the people out there who are less fortunate than him. The ones that deserve the chance of drugs like Clozaril, even if it's a very vague chance that it might help will provide hope, something that's very hard to hold onto in all of this.

I'm saying "the end", but I do know that it's not really the end. Of course there will still be problems along the way, but I do think that, now he's on Clozaril, his life will be much better.

Chris said yesterday that it's so wonderful to be feeling better; that things like owning his own car, for instance, don't matter to him and I couldn't help thinking how nice it was to hear a young person saying this, taking into account what a very material world we are all caught up in, myself included.

As I said earlier, people must come to their own conclusions, but there is no doubt in my mind that my sister's prayer was heard and I was purely a vessel used to pass all of this on in order to help others, and I feel privileged to do so. It's helped me to understand that there is no need to feel bitter if bad things happen to us. I know now that people like my son and millions of other people who suffer in this life are here to teach us humility. Finally, I list three things that I pray this book might do.

* I hope it will help other families to hold on to some hope;

* In a small way contribute towards people being tried on drugs, like Clozaril; and

* Provide an insight to help educate people into a very misunderstood condition—Schizophrenia.

Life is so unfair

Christian has been using Blackshots swimming pool for the past nine months. We were really pleased that he had taken it up again. Before he became ill, he loved to go swimming, so, for us, it was a very positive thing. This is about an incident that he was involve in. This is the sequence of events leading up to what happened.

About three months ago, Chris came home from swimming and said that he had joined as a member. When I read the conditions, I realised that he had joined on the Platinum Packet costing £98.00 and it was totally inappropriate for his needs. It allowed you to bring three friends along and gave access to weight training, etc., for which he was not yet ready.

I rang the centre and spoke to a very understanding lady who said that she felt that Chris wasn't really taking in what she was explaining to him. We got talking and she showed an interest in my book, so I posted her a copy of the manuscript on disk. She refunded Christian's money by cheque.

On Saturday 29th September, Chris went swimming as usual. He goes on Friday, Saturday, Sunday and Monday mornings. He has to go in the mornings as he works in the afternoons. When he got home, he said that two of the attendants called him out of the pool and asked why he spent so much time in there, to which he replied, honestly, that he'd had a mental illness and he was trying to build up his muscles. She then said that he was an excellent swimmer and maybe he could get a job there one day.

On Sunday morning I told Paul about it. I also said that I was a bit worried, but Paul accused me of being paranoid. He said perhaps the lady who had my book, had read it and told some of the staff how brave Chris had been and they were just being nice to him because of it. I kept telling myself that he was right; call it mother's intuition, but I still had some nagging doubts.

The following Friday, 5th September, around 11.30am, Chris rang me at work, very distressed. It was hard to understand what he was saying. An attendant had again called him out of the pool where there were two uniformed police officers waiting to talk to him. One was a sergeant, who began to question him about why he was in there when there were children swimming. Chris said he was running on about children in the showers. I was so cold and I didn't even understand what he was talking about.

I broke down as I realised that I was right to have been worried. I work in an all glass reception office and some of the staff kept asking me what was wrong. I couldn't even answer them as I felt it was too horrendous to talk about. Paul picked me up as soon as I rang him. By the time we got to the leisure centre, we were both in tears. The manager and a young girl who he said was the duty officer met us. Paul was so upset and the manager kept saying that he was only doing his job. I think if Chris had been questioned about anything else, we could have coped.

From there we went to the police station and the young sergeant who had seen Chris, openly admitted that he didn't know the first thing about mental illness. It then transpired that some school teachers had noticed that Chris was in there when the children were swimming, as were a few other men. The deputy head had insisted that the manager have a word with Chris. She told us that she had 75 children under her care and that it was her duty to see that they were protected.

We said, 'Yes of course, we could see where she was coming from. Our sons were small once and we felt the same, but by the same token, so do people who suffer from disabilities'. Readers will remember the poem, 'No Props'. Looking at Chris you would never know that he was ill.

So, it seems that, not only do we have to cope with the onslaughts of this illness, but also the sheer humiliation of incidents such as this. Can you even begin to imagine the outcry if this had happened to someone in a wheelchair. I really wish I had spoken to the pool manager when I first felt uneasy. It probably would not have saved Chris from a lot of distress, but it does take us back to the very real need for education.

I'm still wary about who I talk to as there is still this dreadful stigma. Only a few weeks ago, I found myself responding to several letters in our local paper objecting very strongly to having mentally afflicted persons living near them because of the danger to their everyday lives. Christian was looking forward to being rehoused in this project. Again he rang me at work after reading the letters, asking me why the people didn't want him living near them. One of the residents seems to have thought of a name for the flats already, 'The Nut House' and this is before the roof has even gone on.

So, the swimming pool incident was just another painful experience for us, but most of all for Chris. The police were very good and even came to my house to speak to Chris. The young sergeant is currently reading my manuscript to improve his knowledge of mental illness. I have since received an apology, two free swimming vouchers from the pool and a letter from the police explaining their part in the matter. I do not feel the fault lies with them, or with the head teacher, but the pool manager needs to rethink his policies, as all Chris was doing was swimming. Instead of just having a word with Chris, he rang the child protection team who advised him to call the police. He told us that he had no idea that his staff had spoken to Chris the week before, so he should at least try to improve communications within his organisation.

Paul and I worked very hard to build up Christian's confidence to allow him to go back to the pool, as he kept saying that he felt humiliated. We explained that it wasn't him who should be feeling bad. Yet again, we feel proud of him for having the courage to go back. Not only was this discrimination, but we feel it was also defamation of character. It did affect Chris. In fact, I had to ring Ward 12 on the following evening, as some of his symptoms were returning. The desperate need for public education is all too apparent.

Try to imagine what it must feel like, first, to know that the flat you had been looking forward to moving into for the past four years has been named 'The Nut House' before you've even moved in and, second, you are put through an ordeal such as this for no reason. What is of major concern is that this could have been a young person who had no support and no family and, therefore, no-one with whom to share such a dreadful experience, and who knows what the outcome would have been.

The good news is that I've received a letter from social services after making a formal complaint about this incident, stating that it has been decided that training will now be offered to leisure centres in the hope that it will improve their understanding of mental illness.

It seems so very strange that this should happen just as the book is about to be published, but looking back to all that has happened, is it so very strange? Or is it something that was meant to happen along with all the other things that have happened over the past ten years. Thus, this is another chapter that will warn others about the dreadful things that can happen, if you are unfortunate enough to develop a mental illness. I would like to thank my publisher for allowing me to include this in the book.

Why is this life so unfair?

It's the worst thing that's ever happened
My feelings are hard to explain
So I'll get it all down now on paper
To try to get rid of the pain

Chris had gone swimming as usual
He rang me at work with his fears
Mum, something terrible has happened
Yet another day destined for tears

They called me out of the pool
Two policemen were waiting for me
They kept asking me horrible questions
For the life of me I couldn't see
What they were talking about
Their questions just didn't make sense
I didn't know how to answer
I was feeling so cold and so tense

He kept running on about children
And why I went swimming a lot
He mentioned kids in the showers
What did he mean, tell me what
I'd only gone for a swim
It's far better than lying in bed
I can't get to grips with it all
It keeps going round in my head

We're relieved that he didn't quite grasp it
The injustice too painful to bear
The sadness of this situation
God, why is this life so unfair?

Printed in the United Kingdom by
Lightning Source UK Ltd., Milton Keynes
142656UK00001B/116/A